Dec 4, 1992

To
Dr. Larry
with compliments
of
J. Pinkus

United States
Department of
Agriculture

Agricultural
Research
Service

Agriculture
Handbook
Number 651

An Atlas of Protozoan Parasites in Animal Tissues

C.H. Gardiner
R. Fayer
J.P. Dubey

Abstract

Gardiner, C.H., R. Fayer, and J.P. Dubey.   1988.
An atlas of protozoan parasites in animal tissues.   U.S.
Department of Agriculture, Agriculture Handbook No.
651, 83 p.

This atlas illustrates protozoan parasites in animal
tissues. To facilitate identification, it provides a brief
description of parasites, hosts, transmission, and
pathogenesis of the most important protozoans and
simplified life-cycle drawings. Also included are 257
color photographs of protozoans and associated
lesions, recorded using optimal conditions for identification, and 36 color photomicrographs of fungi that
are commonly confused with protozoans.

KEYWORDS: *Acanthamoeba, Akiba, Anaplasma,
Babesia, Balantidium, Besnoitia, Calyptospora,
Caryospora, Cryptosporidium, Cystoisospora, Cytaux-
zoon, Ehrlichia, Eimeria, Encephalitozoon, Entamoeba,
Frenkelia, Giardia, Glugea, Haemogregarina,
Haemoproteus, Hammondia, Hepatocystis, Hepatozoon,
Hexamita, Histomonas, Ichthyophthirius, Isospora,
Klossiella, Leishmania, Leucocytozoon, Myxosoma,
Naegleria, Pentatrichomonas, Plasmodium,
Pneumocystis, Sarcocystis, Spironucleus, Theileria, Tox-
oplasma, Trichomonas, Trypanosoma.*

Copies of this publication can be purchased from the
Superintendent of Documents, U.S. Government Printing
Office, Washington, DC 20402.

Microfiche copies can be purchased from the National
Technical Information Service, 5285 Port Royal Road,
Springfield, VA 22161.

Agricultural Research Service has no additional copies
for free distribution.

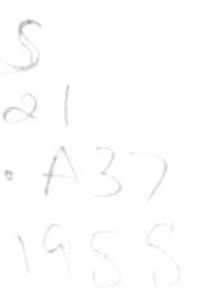

Issued April 1988

Preface

Identification of protozoan parasites in animal tissues is often difficult and confusing. Sometimes it is impossible. There is no single reference containing illustrations of the numerous species of protozoans and their stages as they appear within infected tissues. The intent of this atlas is to fill this void by providing color photomicrographs of these organisms prepared by techniques that best identify them. To further facilitate identification, we have included simplified life-cycle drawings and brief descriptions of the parasites, hosts, transmission, and pathogenesis.

The illustrations in this atlas represent the most common stages under optimal conditions for identification. To obtain them, we have utilized fresh as well as fixed and stained specimens. Most protozoans can be readily identified in tissues stained with hematoxylin and eosin (H&E) and observed with bright field microscopy. Therefore, most illustrations in this atlas show such specimens, and no notation of this stain is made in the legends. Identification of other protozoans is facilitated by special stains, such as Giemsa, Protargol, iron-hematoxylin, periodic acid-Schiff (PAS) reaction, PAS-hematoxylin (PASH), Gram, acid-fast, Gomori methanamine silver, and trichrome, which are noted in the legends. Still other protozoans are best seen by phase contrast or Nomarski interference contrast microscopy or by electron microscopy.

Anaplasma and *Ehrlichia*, historically associated with protozoans but now known to be rickettsiae, are included to aid in differential diagnosis. Because of difficulty in differentiating some fungi from protozoans, several plates have been provided to illustrate those fungi.

Each plate is labeled as color (CP) or black and white (BW) and is numbered sequentially. Each photograph has a plate number followed by a decimal indicating its placement within the plate. Furthermore, nearly every color photo is identified in the legend with a medical illustration number in parentheses. This number references the illustration on file at the Armed Forces Institute of Pathology.

A chart has been included to facilitate identification of coccidian genera, based on the morphology of the sporulated oocysts.

We hope this atlas will aid students, teachers, diagnosticians, and researchers by facilitating identification of protozoan parasites of animals.

Acknowledgments

We express our appreciation to the hundreds of scientists who contributed biological specimens or microscope slides of protozoan parasites to the Registry of Veterinary Pathology, Armed Forces Institute of Pathology, from which many photomicrographs were made.

We also express appreciation to the following associates who provided tissues, mounted specimens, transparencies, or information: P.C. Beaver, Tulane University, New Orleans, LA; R.J. Cawthorne, Regional Veterinary College, Prince Edward Island, Canada; M.L. Eberhard, Delta Regional Primate Center, Covington, LA; J.V. Ernst, Animal Parasitology Institute, Beltsville, MD; P.R. Fitzgerald, University of Illinois, Urbana, IL; J.K. Frenkel, University of Kansas Medical Center, Kansas City, KS; P.C.C. Garnham, London School of Tropical Medicine and Hygiene, Ascot, England; W.J. Hartley, Wallaceville Agricultural Research Center, Upper Hutt, New Zealand; G.D. Imes, Armed Forces Institute of Pathology, Washington, DC; R.G. Leek, Animal Parasitology Institute, Beltsville, MD; N.D. Levine, University of Illinois, Urbana, IL; D.S. Lindsay, Auburn University, Auburn, AL; R.C. Neafie, Armed Forces Institute of Pathology, Washington, DC; R.M. Overstreet, Gulf Coast Research Laboratory, Ocean Springs, MS; M. Rommel, Institute for Parasitology of the Hannover Veterinary College, Hannover, Federal Republic of Germany; L.T. Sangster, Veterinary Diagnostic Laboratory, Tifton, GA; C.A. Speer, Montana State University, Bozeman, MT; R.S. Wacha, Drake University, Des Moines, IA; and R.G. Yaeger, Tulane University, New Orleans, LA.

We thank R.B. Ewing, Animal Parasitology Institute, Beltsville, MD, for the life-cycle drawings and J.E. Luscavage, Armed Forces Institute of Pathology, Washington, DC, for the photomicrographs of most of the specimens.

Contents

Color plates

Black and white plates

An Atlas of Protozoan Parasites in Animal Tissues

By C.H. Gardiner, R. Fayer, and J.P. Dubey[1]

Protozoans are unicellular animals. Most are very small (10-20 μm in diameter), many are somewhat larger (100-200 μm). Even though they are unicellular, some stages in their life cycle may appear multicellular, such as a cyst of *Sarcocystis*, a megaloschizont of *Leucocytozoon*, and a merocyst of *Hepatocystis*. Life cycles are often intricate. They may involve one, two, or more hosts; vectors may be necessary for their spread; and many sizes or shapes of organisms may be present.

The following annotated classification[2] includes only the protozoans in this atlas.

Subkingdom Protozoa
   Phylum Sarcomastigophora—flagella or
      pseudopodia
      Subphylum Mastigophora—flagella in
         trophozoites
         Class Zoomastigophorea—no chromato-
            phores
            Order Kinetoplastida—kinetoplast
               Family Trypanosomatidae—body typi-
                  cally leaflike but may be rounded
                  Genus *Leishmania*
                  Genus *Trypanosoma*
              Order Diplomonadida—bilaterally sym-
                metrical, two similar nuclei
               Family Hexamitidae—body bilaterally sym-
                  metrical, six to eight flagella
                  Genus *Spironucleus* (syn., *Hexamita*)
                  Genus *Giardia*
               Order Trichomonadida—four to six flagella,
                one trailing, no cysts
               Family Trichomonadidae—undulating
                  membrane, trailing flagellum, costa
                  present
                  Genus *Trichomonas*
               Family Monocercomonadidae—costa
                  absent, recurrent flagellum free
                  Genus *Histomonas*

      Subphylum Sarcodina—locomotion by
         pseudopodia
         Superclass Rhizopodea—pseudopodia, not
            axopods
             Order Amoebida—naked, no shell
                Family Vahlkampfiidae—nuclear division by
                  promitosis, flagella may be present
                  Genus *Naegleria*
               Family Hartmannellidae—nuclear division
                  not promitotic, flagellum absent
                  Genus *Acanthamoeba*
              Family Endamoebidae—no flagella, typical-
                  ly in digestive tract
                  Genus *Entamoeba*
   Phylum Microspora—spores of unicellular origin,
      with or without polar filaments
      Class Microsporididea—elongated, oval to tubular
         spores
         Order Pleistophoridida—uninucleate spores
            Family Pleistophoridae—in sporogony, vari-
              able number of sporoblasts form
              Genus *Encephalitozoon*
   Phylum Myxozoa—spores of multicellular origin, with
      two or more polar filaments parasitize poikilo-
      therm vertebrates or annelids
      Class Myxosporea—spore with one or two sporo-
         plasms and one to six polar capsules, mainly
         in fish
         Order Bivalvulida—spores open in two valves
            Family Myxosomatidae—spore circular or pyri-
              form
             Genus *Myxosoma*
   Phylum Ciliophora—cilia or ciliary organelles in at
      least one stage
      Subphylum Rhabdophora—ciliary crown around
         cytostome
      Class Litostomatea—monokinetids with tan-
         gential transverse ribbon cilia present in
         only two orders
         Subclass Trichostomatia—no oral toxicysts
           Family Balantidiidae—cytostome and oral
              cavity long, body cilia holotrichous
              Genus *Balantidium*
      Subphylum Cyrtophora—ciliates with varied
         kinetids
      Class Oligohymenophorea
         Subclass Hymenostomatia—usually holo-
           trichous
           Order Hymenostomatida—body kinetome
              has preoral structure
              Family Ichthyophthiriidae—watchglass
                organelle near buccal cavity
                Genus *Ichthyophthirius*

[1] C.H. Gardiner, Registry of Veterinary Pathology, Armed Forces Institute of Pathology, Washington, DC 20306, and R. Fayer and J.P. Dubey, Animal Parasitology Institute, Beltsville Agricultural Research Center, Beltsville, MD 20705.

The opinions or assertions contained herein are the private views of the authors and are not to be construed as official or as necessarily reflecting the views of the Department of the Navy, the Department of Defense, or the Department of Agriculture.

[2] Modified from Lee, J.J., S.H. Hutner, and E.C. Bovee, "An Il-lustrated Guide to the Protozoa," Society of Protozoologists, The Allen Press, Lawrence, KS, 1985.

Phylum Apicomplexa—motile stage with apical complex

Class Sporozoasida—stage with simple resistant spore (for morphologic characteristics of genera, see chart, p. 20), sexual reproduction

Order Eucoccidiorida—asexual and sexual phases

Family Klossiellidae—monoxenous, microgametes without flagella

Genus *Klossiella*

Family Haemogregarinidae—heteroxenous, in circulatory system of verterbrates, in digestive tract of invertebrates

Genus *Haemogregarina*

Genus *Hepatozoon*

Family Eimeriidae—monoxenous, typically in intestinal epithelial cells, sporogony outside

Genus *Eimeria*

Genus *Isospora*

Genus *Caryospora* (atypical)

Family Cryptosporidiidae—monoxenous, in microvillar border, sporulation inside or outside of host, oocysts with four naked sporozoites

Genus *Cryptosporidium*

Family Sarcocystidae—heteroxenous, producing oocysts with two sporocysts in intestine of definitive host, asexual stages in intermediate host

Genus *Toxoplasma*

Genus *Cystoisospora*

Genus *Besnoitia*

Genus *Hammondia*

Genus *Sarcocystis*

Genus *Frenkelia*

Family Calyptosporidae—heteroxenous, invertebrate intermediate host, definitive hosts poikilothermic

Genus *Calyptospora*

Family Plasmodiidae—heteroxenous, zoite motile, sporozoites naked

Genus *Haemoproteus*

Genus *Leucocytozoon*

Genus *Hepatocystis*

Genus *Plasmodium*

Family Babesiidae—probably no sexual reproduction

Genus *Babesia*

Family Theileriidae—erythrocytic stages smaller than Babesiidae

Genus *Theileria* (syn., *Cytauxzoon*)

Protozoan of undetermined taxonomic status

Genus *Pneumocystis*

Sarcomastigophora

Leishmania

Different species of *Leishmania* occur in the skin, mucous membranes, and visceral organs. Some are found in man, dog, and other mammals; others are in reptiles.

Leishmania spp. are transmitted to mammalian hosts by sandflies (for example, *Lutzomyia* spp. and *Phlebotomus* spp.). During their feeding, the promastigote stage is introduced into the dermis of the mammal and promastigotes are engulfed by histiocytes. Within histiocytes they lose their flagellum, divide, become amastigotes, and continue to divide. Sandflies become infected by ingesting histiocytes containing amastigotes.

Leishmania spp. multiply in macrophages in skin, mucous membranes, and visceral organs, leading to ulceration, eczema, emaciation, and anemia. In visceral leishmaniasis, the spleen is enlarged and the diagnosis can be made by demonstration of organisms in spleen pulp or bone marrow smears.

In tissue section, amastigotes are spherical to ovoid and measure 2 by 5 μm. Each amastigote contains a round nucleus and a rod-shaped kinetoplast. In histologic sections stained with H&E, both structures stain blue (CP1.2). In Giemsa-stained smears, however, the nucleus is red (CP1.1).

Trypanosoma

Two of the main species of cyclically transmitted *Trypanosoma* found in mammals are *T. brucei* and *T. cruzi T. brucei* is transmitted to the mammalian host by tsetse flies. During feeding of the fly, the metacyclic stage is introduced into the circulation of the mammal, where it divides to produce trypomastigotes. A tsetse fly becomes infected by ingesting trypomastigotes that must undergo cyclic development in the fly before becoming infective for another mammalian host. *T. cruzi* is transmitted to mammals by reduviid bugs. While bugs are feeding, the metacyclic form is deposited in bug feces on the mammalian skin. The metacyclic form enters the bloodstream through breaks in the skin and finds its way to the cardiac muscle, where it may transform into an epimastigote or amastigote.

Clinical signs and lesions vary greatly depending on the host and the species of *Trypanosoma*. For example, *T. vivax* and *T. congolense*, which are confined to the plasma, primarily cause anemia, whereas *T. brucei,* which occurs both in the plasma and intercellular tissue and body fluids, can cause anemia as well as

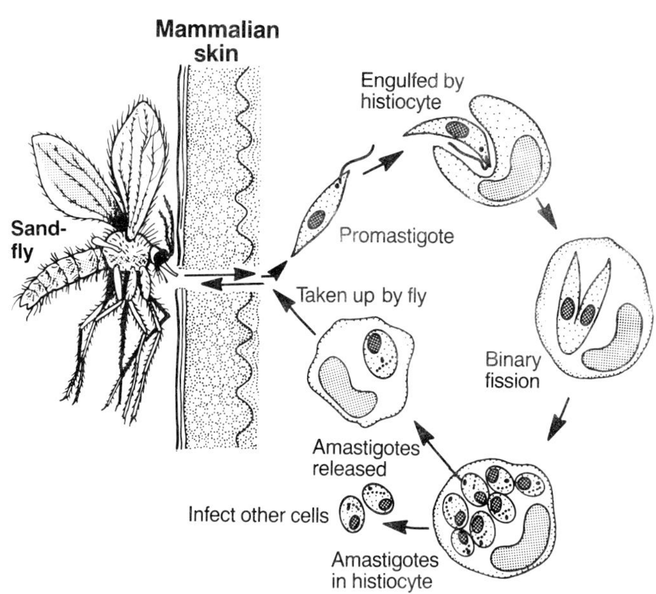

Leishmania

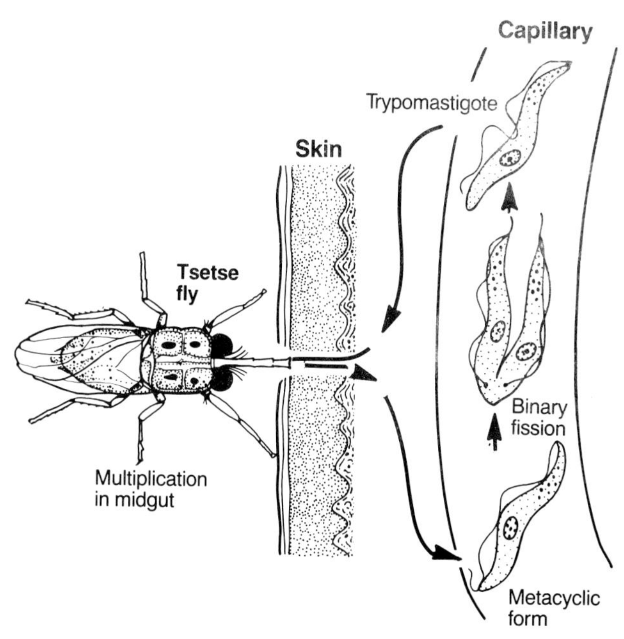

Trypanosoma

degenerative, necrotic, and inflammatory changes. *T. cruzi* causes myocarditis and megacolon.

Trypomastigotes are polymorphic but most often are elongate and have a flagellum with associated undulating membrane (CP1.3, 1.4). In Giemsa-stained blood smears, trypomastigotes of *T. cruzi* can be differentiated from those of *T. brucei* because the former have a larger kinetoplast and are commonly crescent shaped, whereas trypomastigotes of other *Trypanosoma* species have a smaller kinetoplast and are seldom crescent shaped. *T. cruzi* is the only member of the genus to have an amastigote form in its life cycle. Collections of amastigotes are usually found in pseudocysts (CP1.5). *T. cruzi* is usually larger than the *Leishmania* spp. The kinetoplast of *T. cruzi* is larger

and much more basophilic when stained with H&E than that of the *Leishmania* spp. (CP1.6). Trypomastigotes of other species of *Trypanosoma* can be found in a wide range of hosts, such as snakes, frogs, and birds.

T. evansi, T. equinum, and *T. equiperdum* are transmitted mechanically, the first two by biting flies and the last one through coitus. The only stage found in these trypanosomes is the trypomastigote.

T. evansi affects a wide range of hosts. It causes serious illness (called surra) in horses, camels, buffaloes, and oxen. Edema and emaciation are the most prominent signs. *T. equinum* and *T. equiperdum* chiefly affect equids.

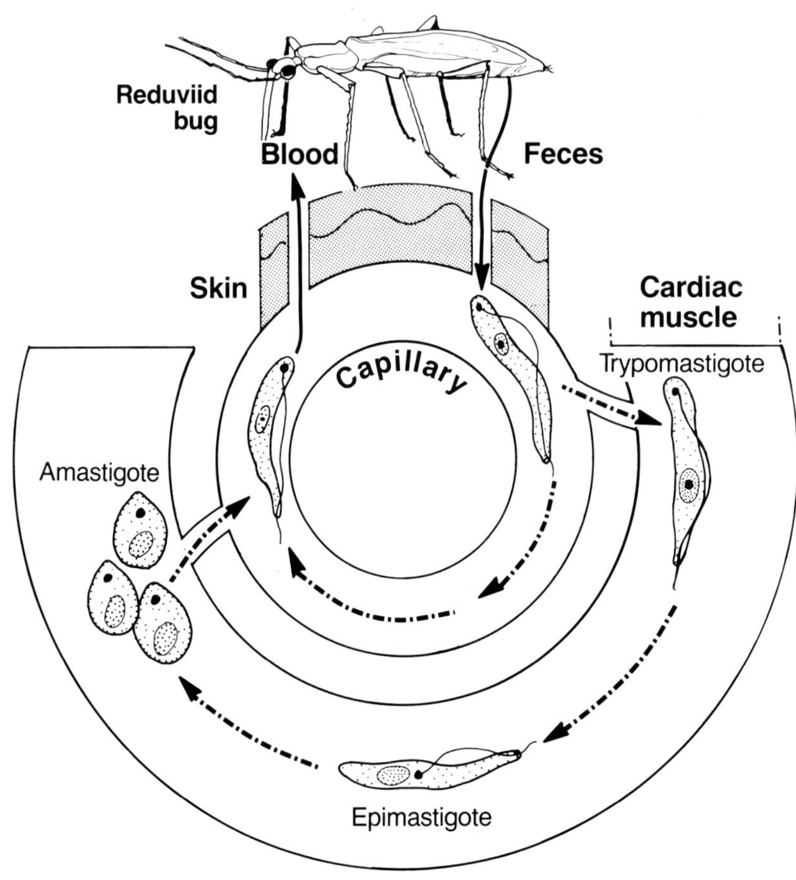

Trypanosoma cruzi

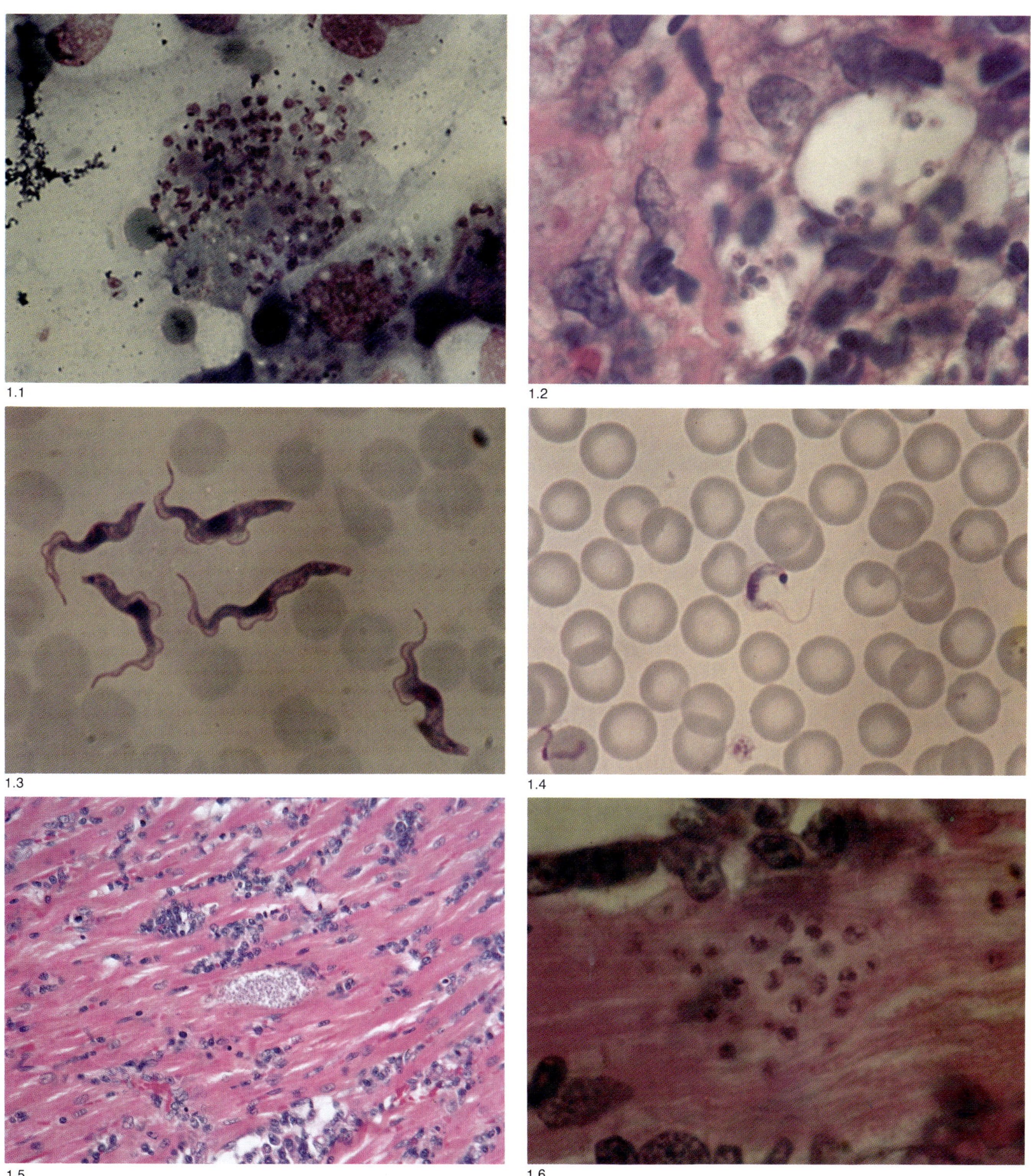

Color plate 1.—*Leishmania* spp. and *Trypanosoma* spp. of animals: 1.1, Spleen imprint from dog with numerous amastigotes of *L. donovani* ruptured from macrophage, X 1500, Giemsa stain (84-9338). 1.2, Dermis of hamster experimentally infected with *L. braziliensis* and containing amastigotes within vacuoles in macrophages, X 1500 (84-9339). 1.3, Peripheral blood smear from experimentally infected mouse containing trypomastigotes of *T. brucei*, X 1500, Giemsa stain (84-9340). 1.4, Peripheral blood smear from experimentally infected mouse containing trypomastigote of *T. cruzi*, X 1500, Giemsa stain (84-9341). 1.5, Heart of dog with numerous amastigotes (pseudocyst) of *T. cruzi* in myofibril, X 25 (84-5305). 1.6, Heart of dog with amastigotes of *T. cruzi*, each with large, basophilic kinetoplast, X 1500 (84-5306).

Flagellates

Numerous genera and species of flagellated protozoans are found in animals. Most live in the lumen of the intestinal tract. Others live on the gills of fish and some in the urogenital tract. Flagellates have a simple, one-host life cycle. The flagellated stage transforms into a resistant cyst, which is transmitted from one animal to another.

Giardia is the most common flagellate of mammals and birds (CP2.1-2.3). Its trophozoites are binucleate and have four pairs of flagella. Trophozoites adhere to microvilli of epithelial cells of the small intestine. In histologic section, it is often difficult to demonstrate nuclei and flagella, and there is no undulating membrane.

Pentatrichomonas spp. differ from *Giardia* because they have a single nucleus, and one flagellum is attached to the body wall to form an undulating membrane (CP2.4).

Spironucleus (syn., *Hexamita*) sp., another flagellate, is smaller than either *Giardia* or *Pentatrichomonas* and lacks an undulating membrane (CP2.5).

Trichomonas caviae occurs in the intestines of guinea pigs. Its flagella are readily seen in stained fecal smears (CP2.6).

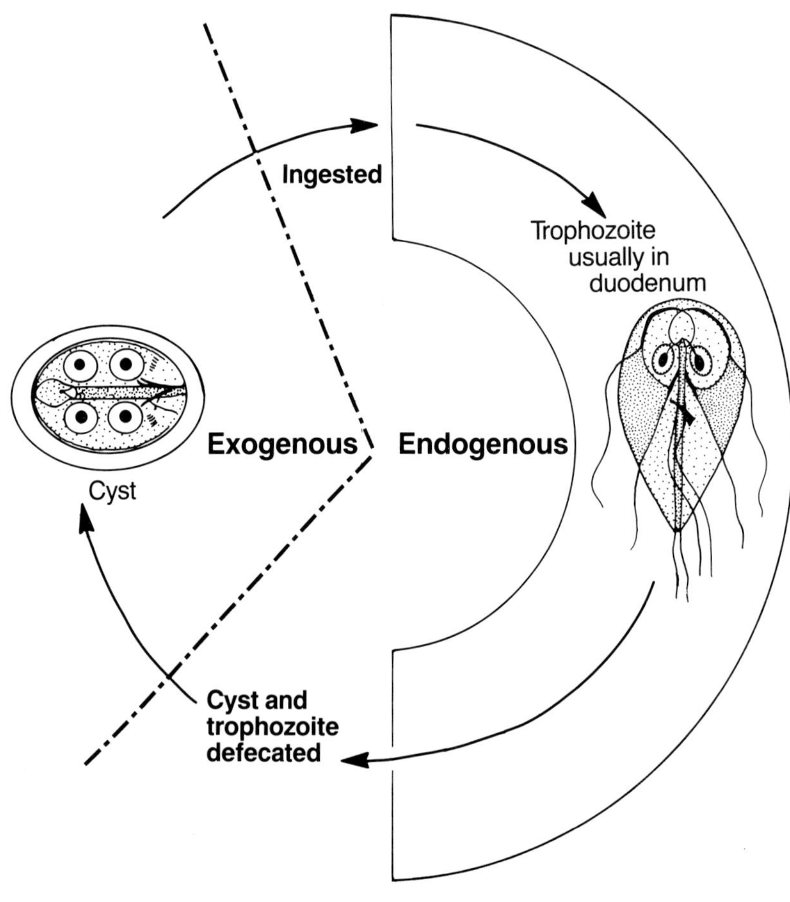

Giardia

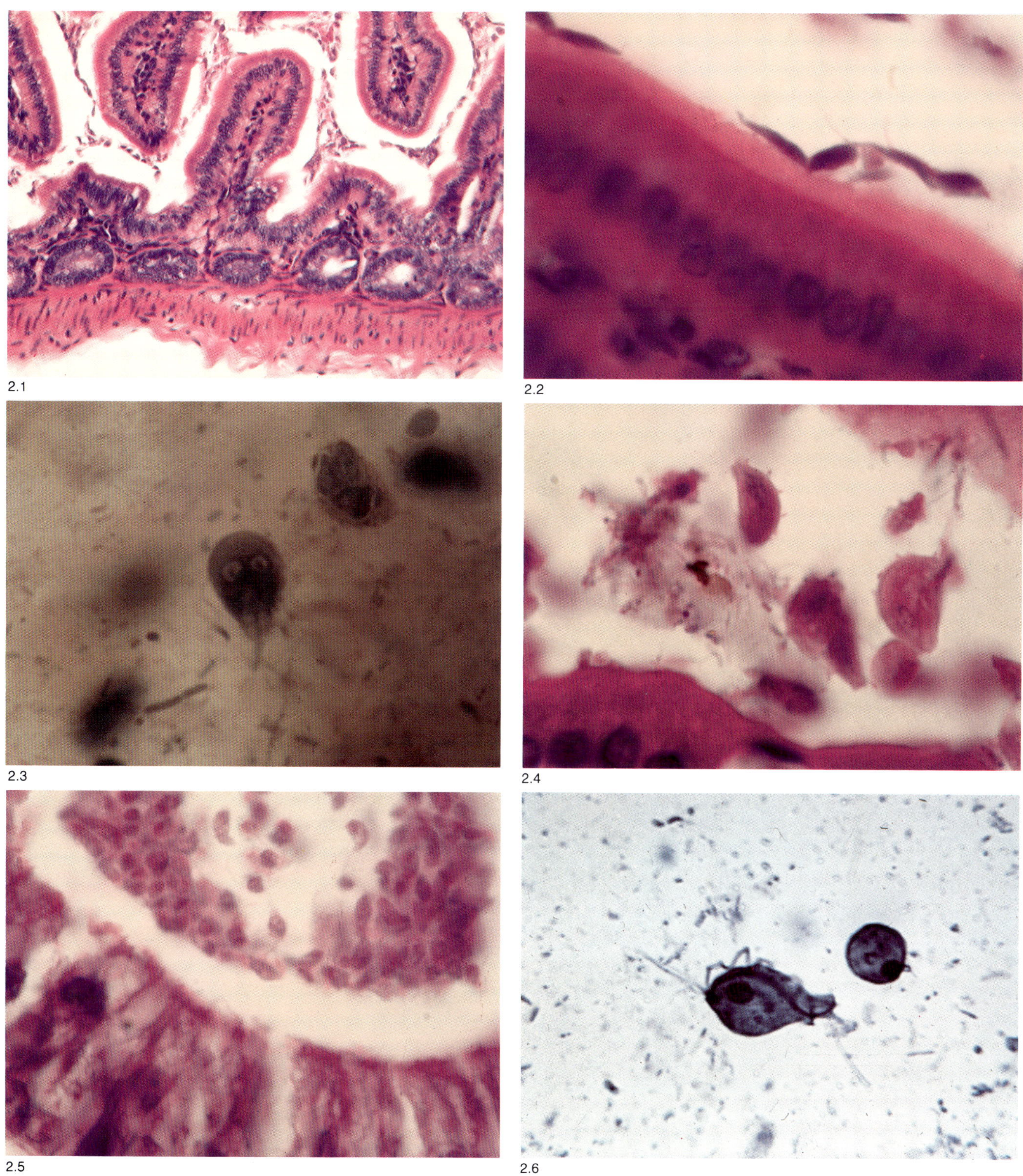

Color plate 2.—Flagellates of animals: 2.1, Small intestine of canary with numerous *Giardia* sp., X 250 (84-9342). 2.2, Higher magnification of trophozoites of *Giardia* sp. attached to intestinal villus of canary, X 1500 (84-9343). 2.3, Human fecal smear containing trophozoite of *G. lamblia* with two nuclei, X 1500, iron-hematoxylin stain (84-9344). 2.4, Lumen of small intestine of hamster containing trophozoites of *Pentatrichomonas* sp. with large nucleus and undulating flagellum, X 1500 (84-9345). 2.5, Large intestine of pigeon containing trophozoites of *Spironucleus* sp. with pyriform shape, X 1500 (84-9346). 2.6, Fecal smear of guinea pig containing trophozoites of *Trichomonas caviae* with undulating membrane and large single nucleus, X 1100, Protargol stain (84-9347).

Histomonas

Histomonas meleagridis affects poultry. Its life cycle is complex. Free trophozoites passed in feces are very delicate and essentially have no role in transmission. Trophozoites within eggs of the roundworm *Heterakis* are readily infective to other birds. Usually heterakid eggs are ingested by earthworms, and birds become infected with both the roundworms and the flagellates after ingesting such earthworms. In the avian intestine, the trophozoite is released from the roundworm egg and invades the cecal wall. It loses its flagellum and becomes very pleomorphic and amoeboid. It often migrates to the liver.

H. meleagridis causes enlarged, rather hemorrhagic ceca and characteristic, depressed liver lesions. In tissues, trophozoites occur in clusters. They vary in size (5-20 μm) and shape and are poorly stained with H&E (CP3.2, 3.5) but stain brilliantly with PAS (CP3.3, 3.4, 3.6).

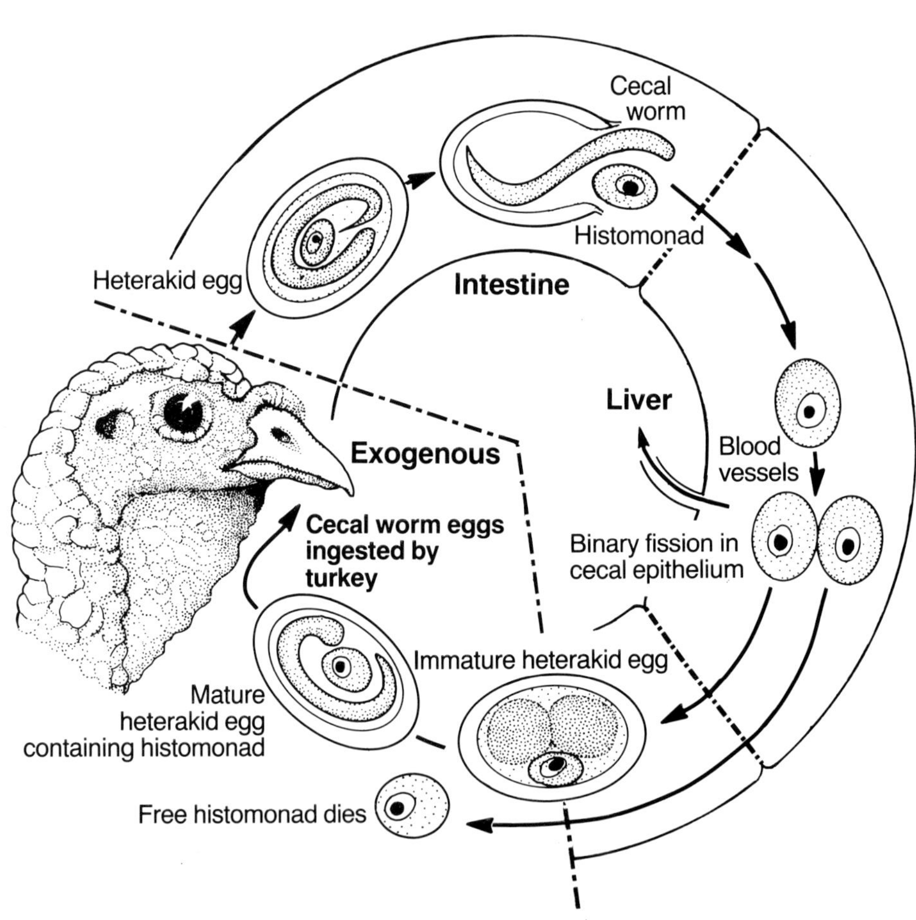

Histomonas

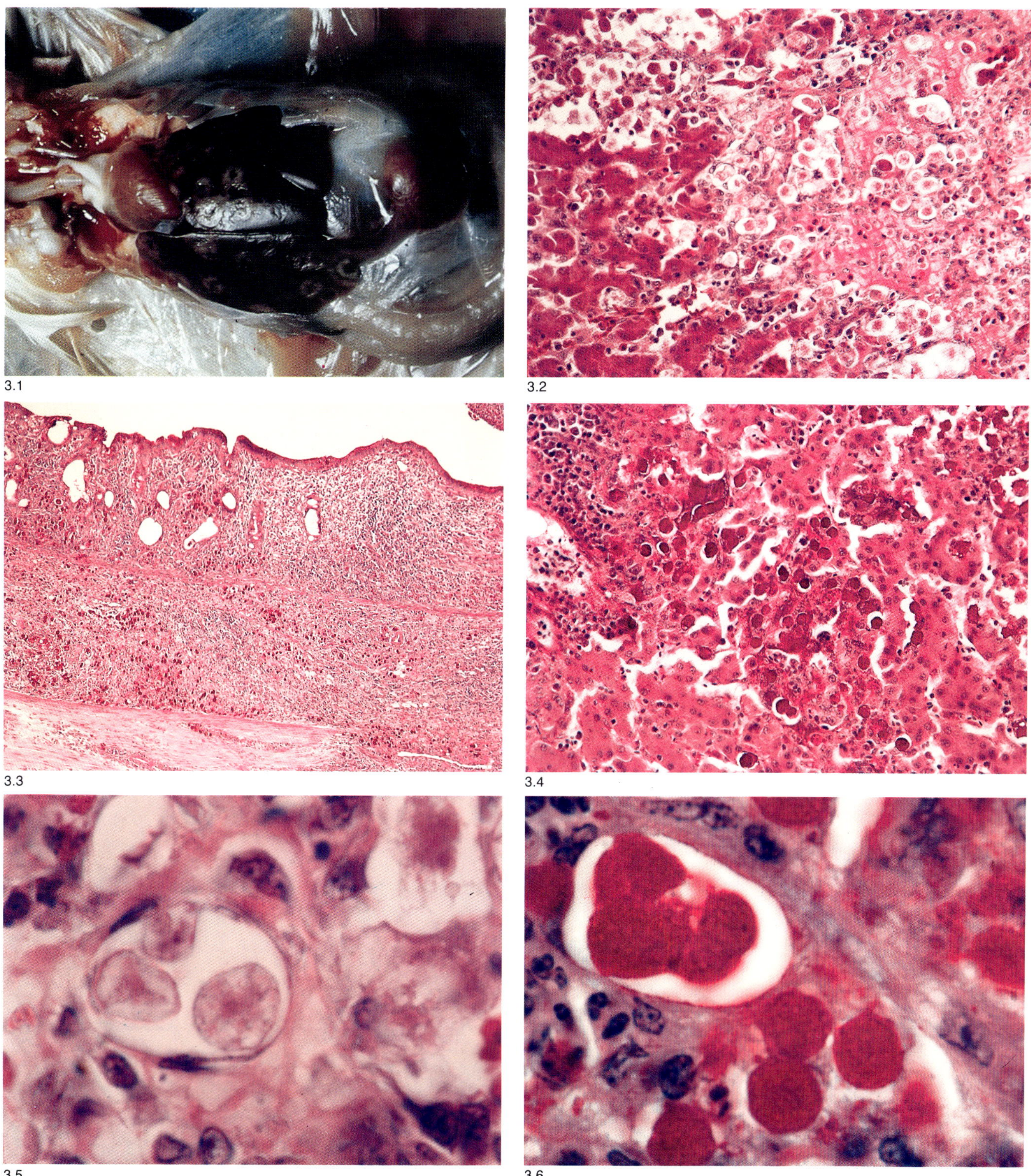

Color plate 3.—*Histomonas meleagridis* of chickens: 3.1, Liver infected with *H. meleagridis* (84-9348).   3.2, Liver infected with *H. meleagridis* and showing hepatic necrosis and faintly stained trophozoites, X 250 (84-9349).   3.3, Cecum infected with *H. meleagridis* and containing trophozoites (red) throughout wall, × 60, PAS stain (84-9350). 3.4, Liver with trophozoites (red) throughout parenchyma, X 250, PAS stain (84-9353). 3.5, Liver with enlarged trophozoites of *H. meleagridis,* X 1500 (84-9351). 3.6, Cecum with enlarged brightly stained trophozoites of *H. meleagridis* in clusters within wall, X 1500, PAS stain (84-9352).

Amoebae

Amoebae include obligate and facultative parasites as well as free-living forms. *Entamoeba* is an important obligate parasite. Its life cycle is direct. Ingestion causes infection and development of trophozoites. The resistant cyst stage is excreted in the feces. Trophozoites reside in the lumen of the intestine and may invade the intestinal wall and other extraintestinal organs. *E. histolytica* and *E. invadens* can be found in the tissues of animals. *E. histolytica* occurs in man but is transmissible to dogs, cats, and other animals. *E. invadens* occurs in reptiles. The nucleus of both has chromatin plaques at the periphery and a small endosome. *E. histolytica* can cause congestion, petechial hemorrhages, and ulcers in the large intestine. In animals, infection is generally confined to the large intestine, but in man it can invade other organs. *E. histolytica* ranges from 15 to 50 μm in "diameter"

(CP4.1, 4.2). *E. invadens* (CP4.3) is smaller (10-35 μm). The cytoplasm of *E. histolytica* is often light staining and granular, whereas the cytoplasm of *E. invadens* often stains darker and is agranular at one pole (CP4.3). Cysts of *Entamoeba* are round and contain one or more chromatoid bodies.

Soil and waterborne free-living amoebae such as *Acanthamoeba* and *Naegleria* can become parasitic. They have a life cycle similar to that of *Entamoeba*. They enter the host accidentally through the mouth or nose and invade the central nervous system via the cribriform plate. They have been found in other organs as well. Both genera have very distinctive nuclei. The nucleus does not have peripheral plaques of chromatin and the endosome is extremely large (CP4.4-4.6). *Naegleria* trophozoites may also have flagella when free-living in water. Both organisms can cause meningoencephalitis.

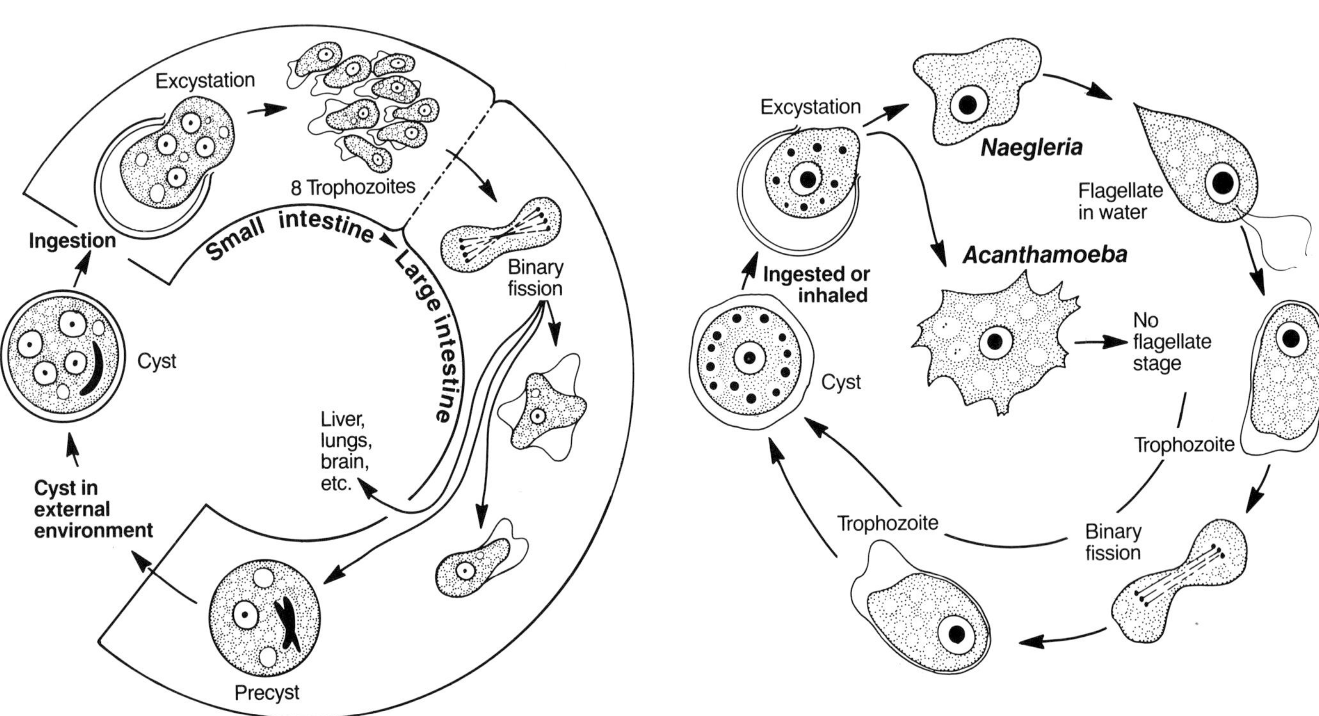

Entamoeba

Acanthamoeba, Naegleria

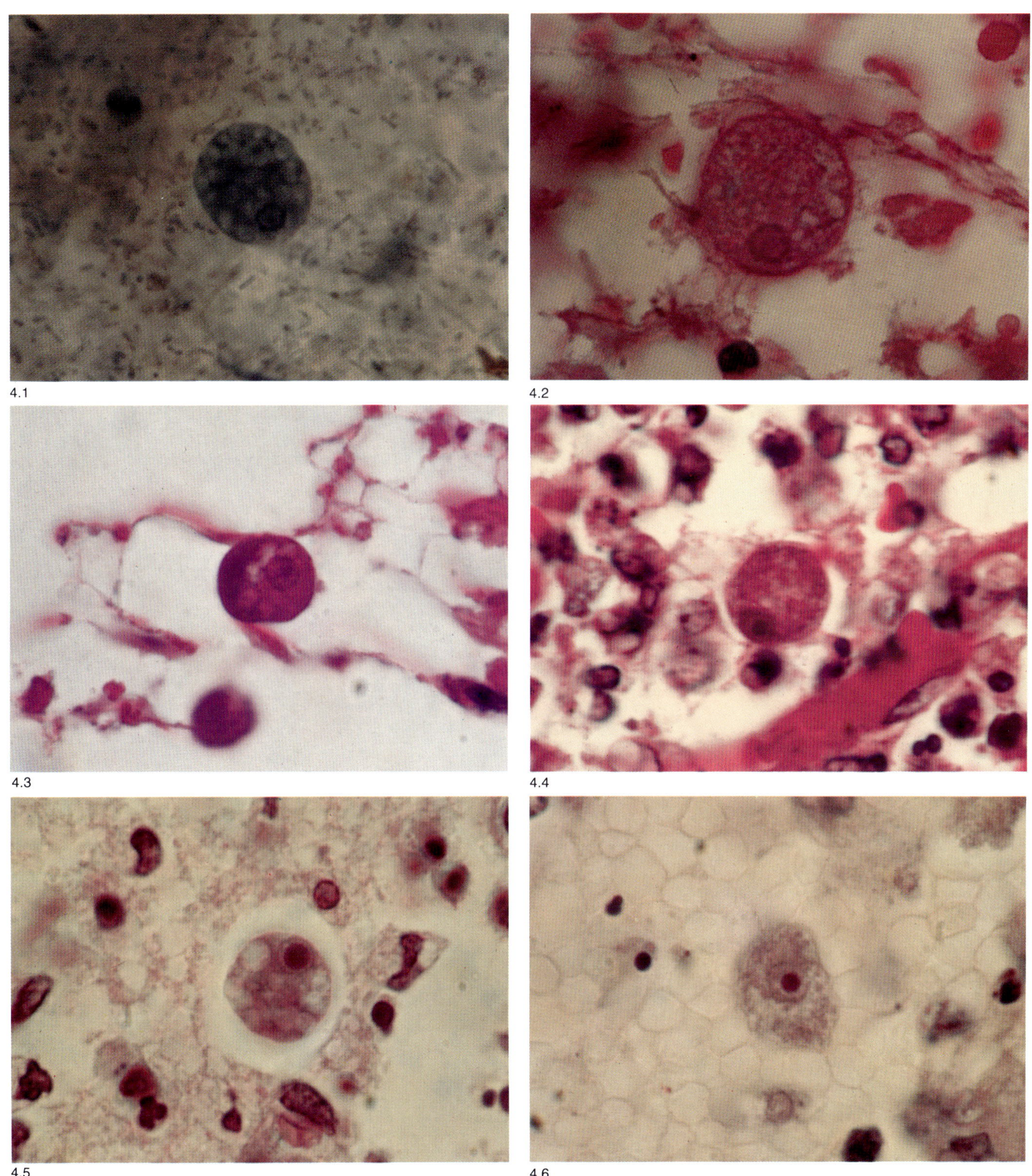

Color plate 4.—Amoebae of animals: 4.1, Human fecal smear containing trophozoite of *Entamoeba histolytica* with small endosome and chromatin plaques at periphery of nucleus, X 1500, iron-hematoxylin stain (84-9354).   4.2, Intestine of monkey with trophozoite of *E. histolytica*, X 1500 (84-9355).   4.3, Small intestine of rattlesnake containing trophozoite of *E. invadens* with small endosome, X 1500 (84-9356).   4.4, Heart of dog containing trophozoite of *Acanthamoeba* sp. with large dark endosome, X 1500 (84-9357).   4.5, Brain of experimentally infected mouse containing trophozoites of *A. culbertsoni* with large endosome, X 1500 (84-9358).   4.6, Brain of experimentally infected monkey containing trophozoite of *Naegleria fowleri* with large endosome, X 1500 (84-9359).

Microspora

Numerous genera of microspora infect animals. *Encephalitozoon* is perhaps the most widely recognized genus, infecting many mammals and a few birds. The genus *Glugea* usually infects fish. Transmission is thought to be direct—by carnivorism—or by spores that pass from the body in urine if the kidney is infected, or spores that may be liberated from tissues when the host dies. When the spore is ingested, the sporont within the spore is liberated and either is engulfed by macrophages or invades endothelial cells, where it undergoes asexual reproduction to form numerous sporoblasts. Sporoblasts round up and secrete a thick, resistant spore wall.

Spores range from 2 to 15 μm in length. Immature spores are often smaller than mature spores (CP5.1, 5.2). Microsporan spores have dark staining annular masses, perhaps due to the coiled filament, which can be demonstrated with a variety of stains (CP5.1-5.3, 5.5). In addition, all stages of microspora are visible with Gram stain (CP5.2, 5.3). Mature spores are acid-fast (CP5.5) and contain a PAS-positive polar granule (CP5.4).

Ultrastructurally the spore has a thick outer coat enclosing a filament and one or two nuclei. One end of the filament is attached to the spore wall and the other end is coiled from 4 to over 30 times depending on the species.

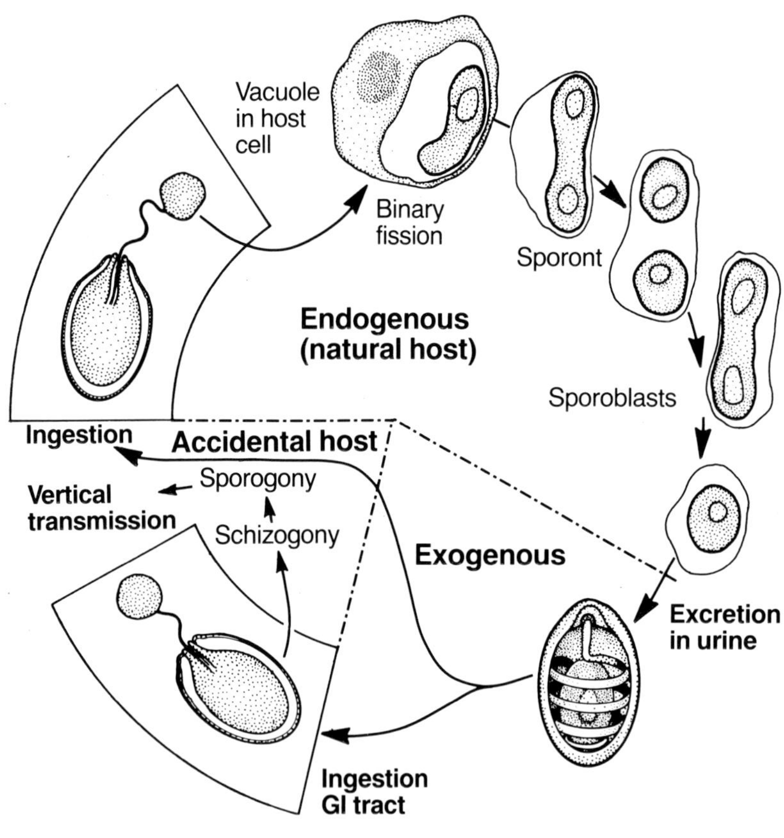

Microspora

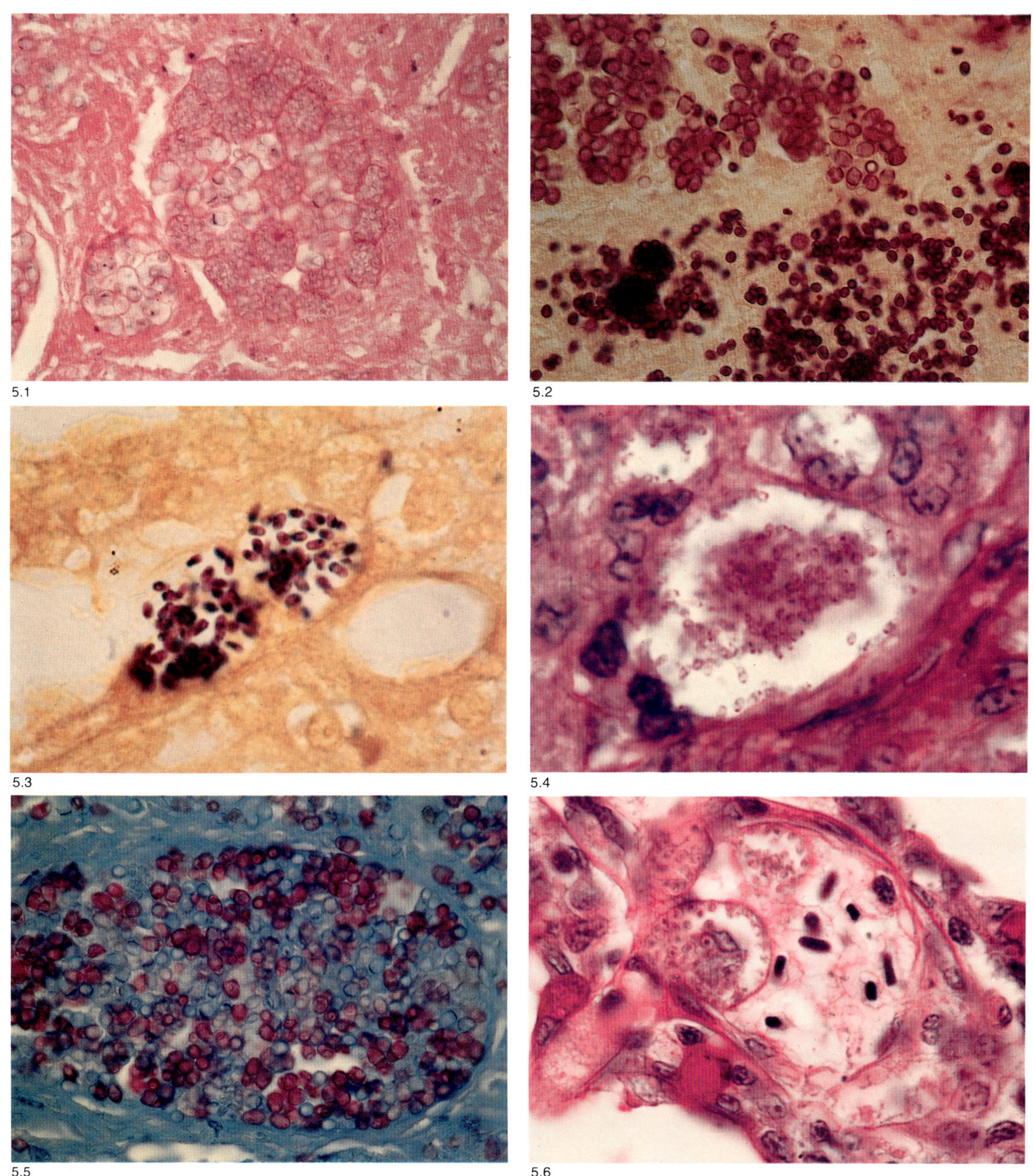

Color plate 5.—Microspora of animals: 5.1, Muscle of garter snake containing immature (smaller) and mature spores with basophilic annular masses, X 630 (84-5273). 5.2, Muscle of garter snake with immature (dark) and mature (lighter) spores of microspora, X 630, Brown and Hopps tissue Gram stain (84-5292). 5.3, Kidney of rabbit with *Encephalitozoon* sp., X 1500, Brown and Hopps tissue Gram stain (84-9360). 5.4, Liver of lovebird with PAS-positive polar granule visible in each spore, X 1500, PAS stain (84-9361). 5.5, Muscle of garter snake with dark-blue stained annular rings and red-stained (acid-fast) mature spores, X 630, Ziehl Nielsen acid-fast stain (84-5276). 5.6, Blood vessel in gill of fish containing numerous microspora within hyperplastic endothelial cells, X 1000, PAS stain (84-9362).

Myxozoa

Myxozoa are found in numerous cold-blooded vertebrates and annelids. Their life cycle is not completely known. Infection begins with ingestion of spores. The motile sporoplasm (amoebula) escapes through the spore coat and penetrates the gut wall. Via the circulation it is carried to extraintestinal tissues. The sporoplasm undergoes asexual division to form a multinucleate sporont, which matures into spores. Masses of spores form myxozoan cysts (CP6.1, 6.2).

Myxosporidia cause several serious diseases of fish, and heavy infections can destroy large numbers of them. The cysts or infiltrations are found in cartilage, muscle, gut wall, gills, brain, skin, and the excretory system.

Spores have varied shapes, from ovoid (CP6.3) to elongate (CP6.5, 6.6). All are multicellular containing two polar capsules (cnidocysts) (CP6.2-6.6), which stain intensely blue with Giemsa. Mature spores are often weakly stained with H&E (CP6.2) but are strongly acid-fast (CP6.4).

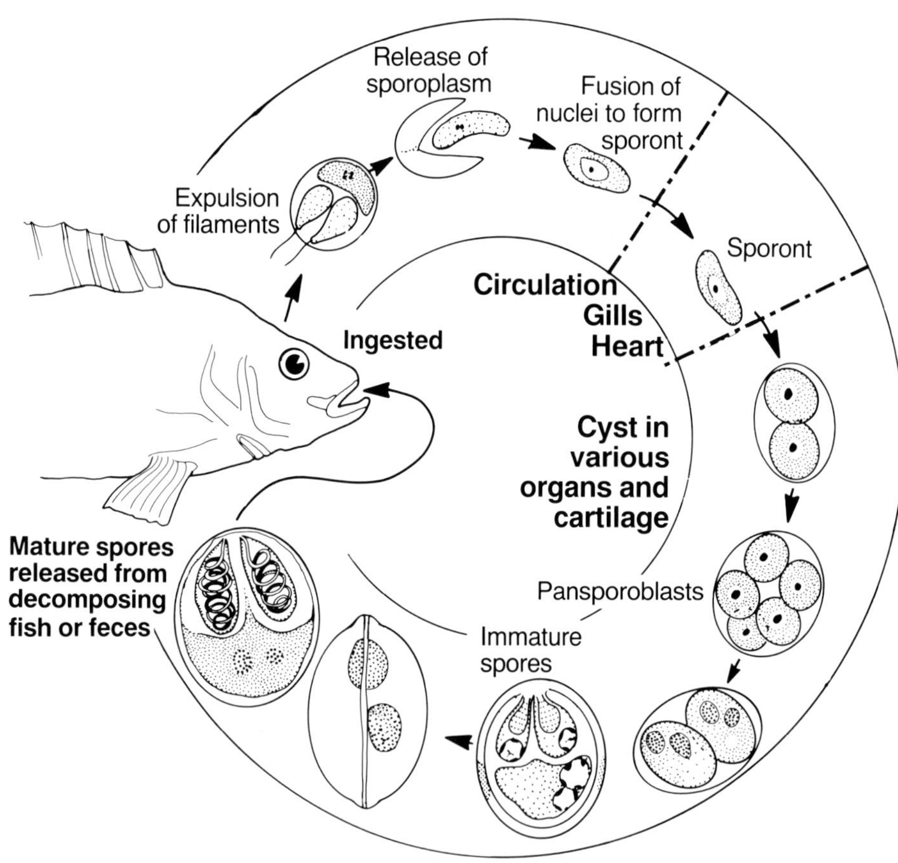

Myxozoa

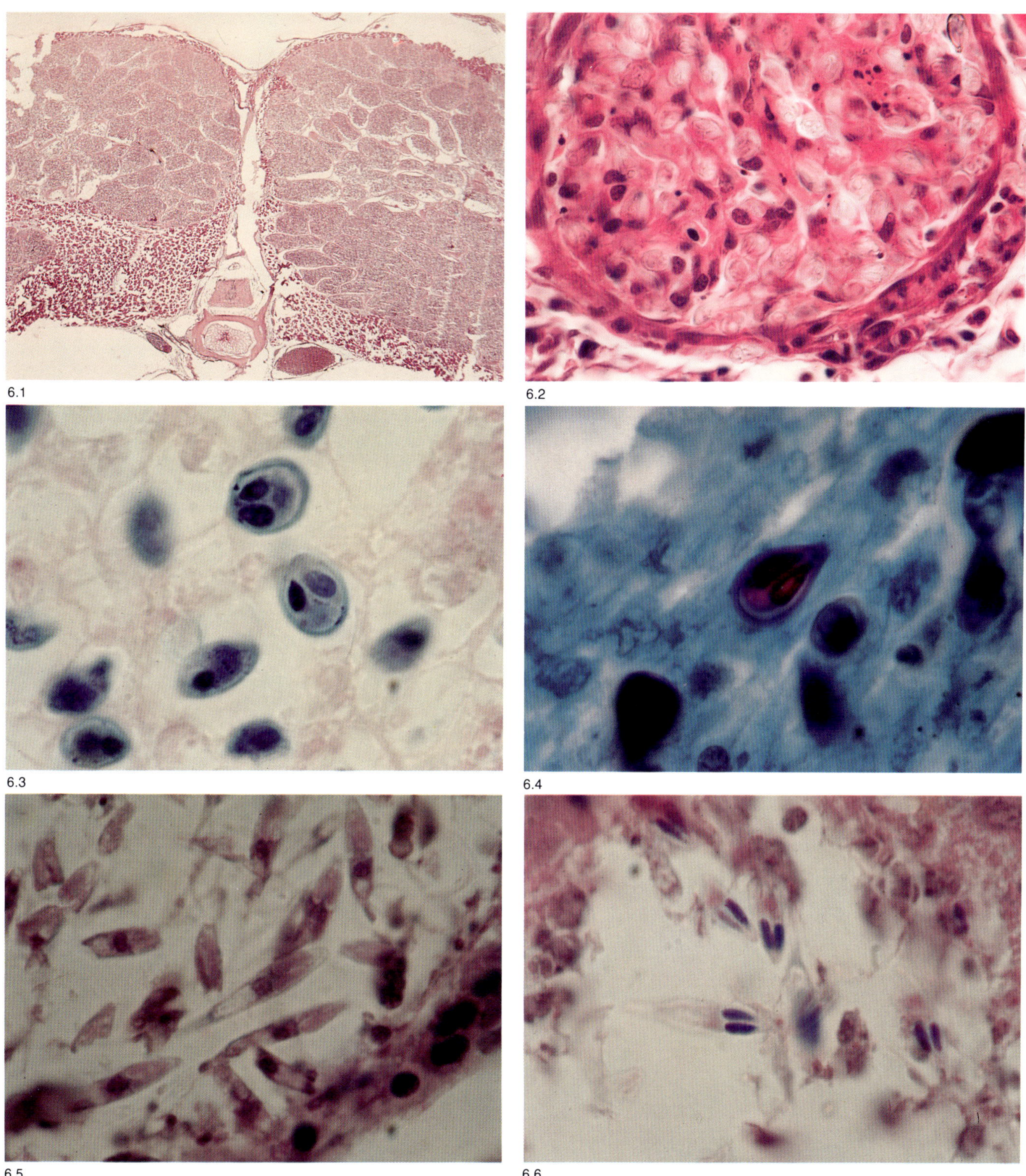

Color plate 6.—Myxozoa of fish: 6.1, Muscle with multiloculate myxozoan cysts, X 15 (84-9363).   6.2, Muscle with refractive spores, X 630 (84-9364).   6.3, Spinal cord containing *Myxosoma cerebralis* with intensely blue polar capsules, X 1500, Giemsa stain (84-9365).   6.4, Spinal cord with acid-fast mature spore of *M. cerebralis,* X 1500, Ziehl Nielsen acid-fast stain (84-9366).   6.5, Gill filament with numerous elongate spores, X 1500 (84-9367).   6.6, Gill filament containing spores with intensely blue polar capsules, X 1500, Giemsa stain (84-9368).

Numerous genera of ciliates are found in the digestive tract of domestic animals. Most have direct life cycles. Cysts passed in the feces are ingested, and the trophozoite is released in the digestive tract, where it undergoes either asexual or sexual multiplication.

Trophozoites have surface cilia. Cilia may be of the same length (CP7.2) or form tufts (CP7.4). When the trophozoites are in tissue, the cilia may not be demonstrable.

Balantidium sp. is a common ciliate in pigs, rodents, and primates. Trophozoites have a kidney-shaped macronucleus and often a contractile vacuole (CP7.2, 7.3). *B. coli* normally occurs in the lumen of the large intestine and is associated with no change in mucosa. Occasionally it invades the mucosa and causes mild to severe enteritis and dysentery.

Though most ciliates are nonpathogenic commensals, often after the host dies, they move to the liver via mesenteric veins or into tissue of the intestinal tract and may be mistaken for pathogens. These ciliates commonly have an elongate nucleus, which is round in cross section (CP7.5).

Ichthyophthirius spp. are pathogens of fish. Trophozoites of *Ichthyophthirius* spp. may penetrate the skin and produce "Ich" or white spot disease. The trophozoites eventually develop a cyst wall, drop off the fish, and enter the water, where they rupture and release trophozoites that reinfect other fish. *Ichthyophthirius* spp. are 75 μm to 1 mm in diameter, are uniformly ciliated, and have a crescent-shaped nucleus (CP7.6).

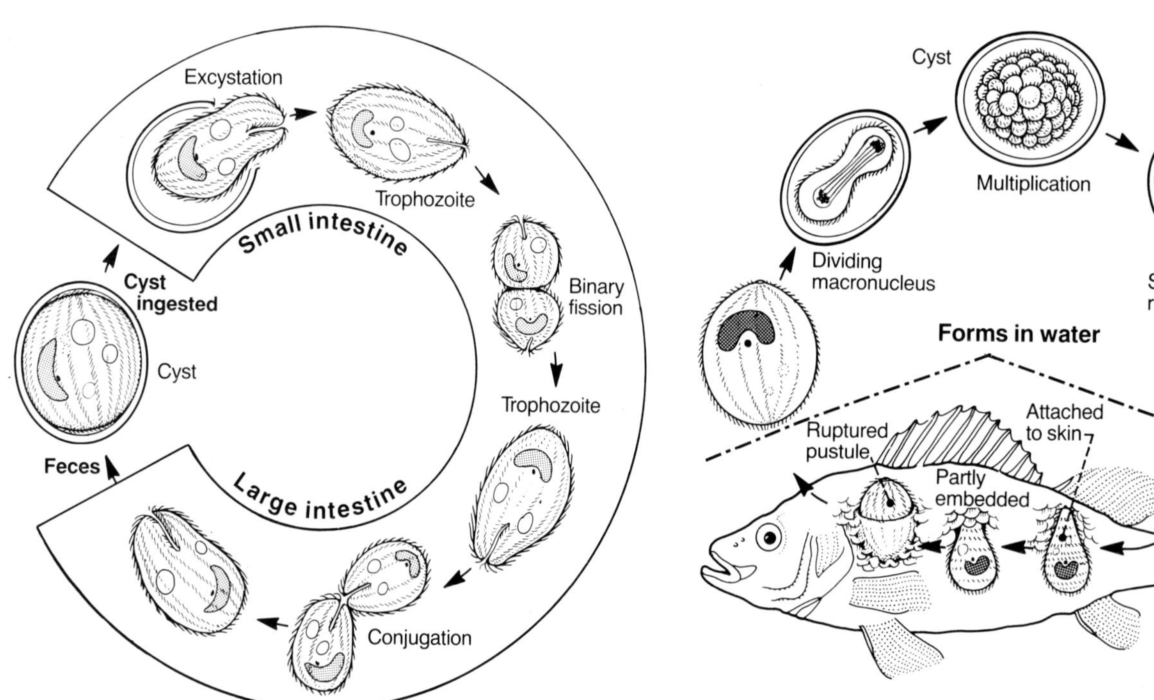

Balantidium

Ichthyophthirius

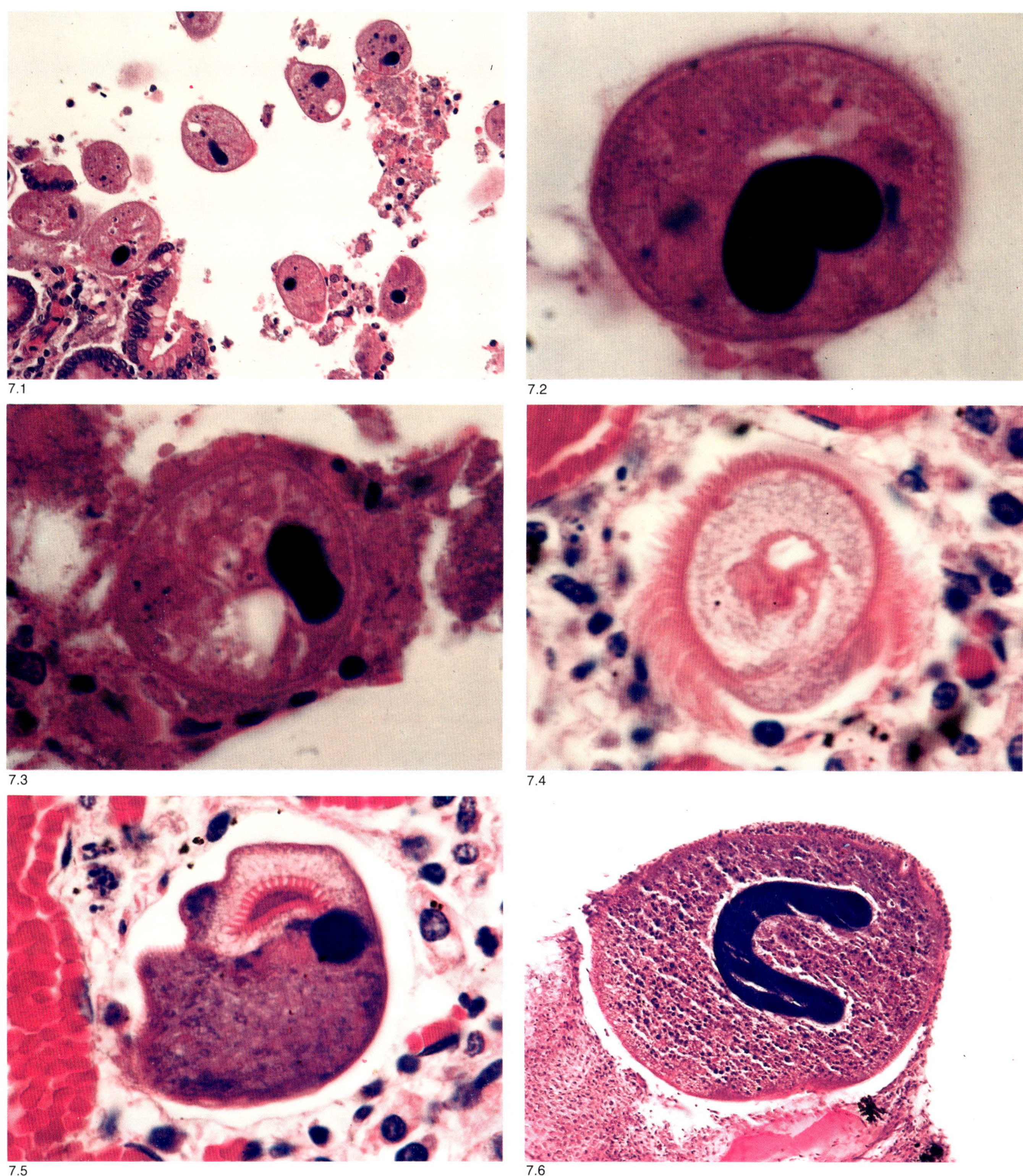

7.1

7.2

7.3

7.4

7.5

7.6

Color plate 7.—Ciliates of animals: 7.1, Large intestine of gorilla containing numerous *Balantidium* sp., X 250 (84-9369). 7.2, Large intestine of gorilla containing *Balantidium* sp. with large macronucleus and distinct cilia, X 1500 (84-9370). 7.3, Lamina propria of large intestine of gorilla containing *Balantidium* sp. with indistinct cilia, prominent basophilic macronucleus, and clear contractile vacuole, X 1000 (84-9371). 7.4, Large intestine of horse containing unidentified ciliate with tufts of cilia, X 1000 (84-9372). 7.5, Large intestine of horse containing unidentified ciliate with large basophilic nucleus and prominent cytostome, X 1000 (84-9373). 7.6, Skin of fish with *Ichthyophthirius* sp., X 160 (84-9374).

The taxonomic status of *Pneumocystis* is unsettled; some workers place it with the protozoa and others with the yeasts. This situation exists because basic questions regarding the biology of this organism, including aspects of its life cycle and transmission, are unanswered. A hypothetical life cycle is presented here as an aid to identification of stages. The terms used to describe these stages are those used for the Apicomplexa.

P. carinii is a common species. The entire life cycle occurs in the lungs of many species of mammals and is direct. Mature cysts rupture, releasing eight intracystic bodies that develop into trophozoites.

Trophozoites copulate or fuse to form a diploid trophozoite, which develops into a precyst, an intermediate form between the trophozoite and cyst in which the number of nuclei increases from one to eight. In the most mature stage of the precyst, each nucleus, a mitochondrion, and some adjacent cytoplasm become surrounded by a limiting membrane. As each of these bodies becomes independent and a thick wall forms around them, the precyst becomes a cyst containing eight intracystic bodies.

Pneumocystis should be regarded as an opportunistic pathogen affecting those humans or animals with impaired immunity. Pathological changes are usually limited to the lungs. On gross examination, the lungs are usually enlarged, are firm, and do not collapse. Cut surfaces appear dry, with irregular gray, brown, or pink areas of consolidation and sometimes contain liquefied foci. Histologically the lung appears solid and highly cellular, with massive mononuclear infiltration, predominantly plasma cells, histiocytes, or lymphocytes. With H&E stain, a characteristic foamy, fine granular, eosinophilic exudate fills the alveolar space, but parasites are poorly stained (CP8.1-8.3).

Pneumocystis stages are best demonstrated with the GMS stain (CP8.4, 8.5). Some are spherical and measure 2-6 μm in diameter, others appear collapsed. Smears from the lungs may contain cysts with up to eight intracystic bodies when stained with Giemsa (CP8.6). Imprints of the lung may show cysts within a foamy matrix.

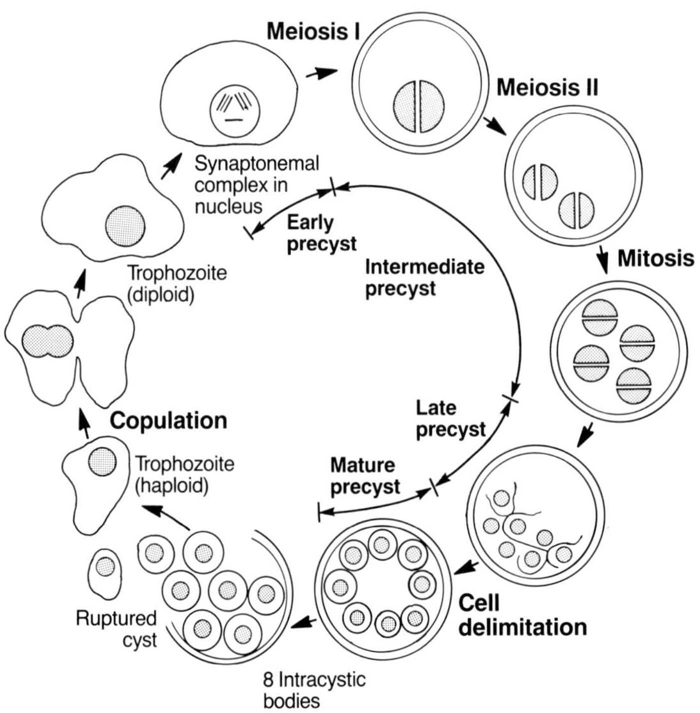

Pneumocystis

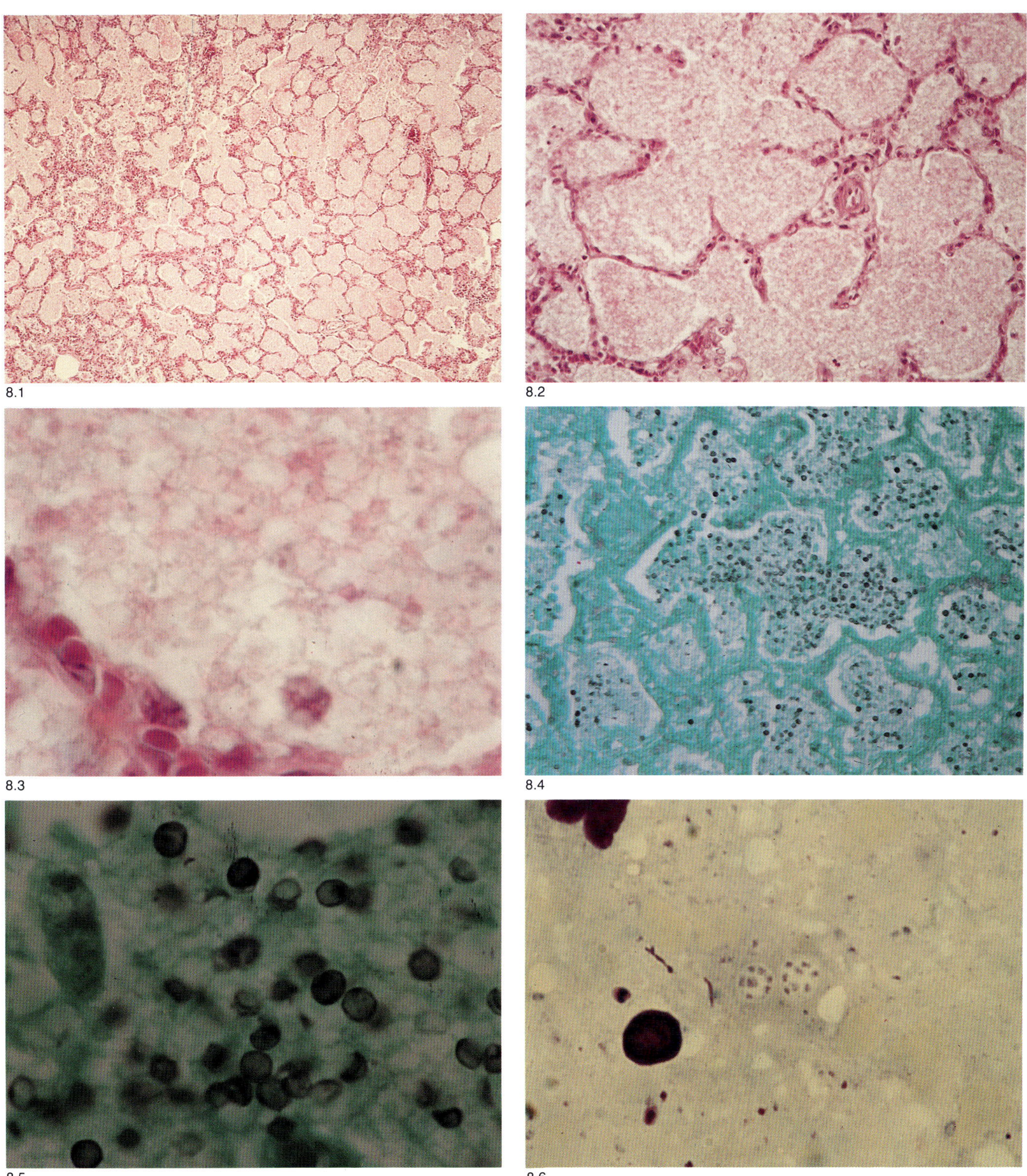

Color plate 8.—*Pneumocystis* sp. of mammals: 8.1, Lung of horse with severe pneumocystosis, X 60 (84-9375). 8.2, Lung of horse at higher magnification showing alveoli filled with foamy eosinophilic material, X 250 (84-9376). 8.3, Lung of horse at very high magnification showing eosinophilic material, X 1500 (84-9377). 8.4, Lung of horse with numerous organisms in alveoli, X 250, Gomori methanamine silver stain (GMS) (84-5303). 8.5, Lung of horse with numerous darkly stained ovoid organisms, X 1500, GMS stain (84-5304). 8.6, Lung smear of rat containing *Pneumocystis* cysts with intracystic organisms, X 1500, Giemsa stain (84-9378).

Apicomplexa

Coccidia in the genera *Cryptosporidium, Eimeria, Isospora, Sarcocystis,* and *Toxoplasma* are the most economically important group of protozoans in domestic animals in the United States. Historically the structure of the sporulated oocyst, especially the number of sporocysts and sporozoites, was used as a major characteristic to differentiate genera of coccidia. The accompanying chart provides a comparative guide to the morphology of sporulated oocysts among these and other genera of coccidia.

Eimeria

Over a thousand species of *Eimeria* are known that primarily infect cells lining the intestine of domestic and wild mammals and birds (CP9-17). The life cycle for each species is host specific and direct. Unsporulated oocysts (BW1.1) are shed in feces and sporulate (BW1.2) in the environment to become infectious. Following ingestion, sporozoites (BW1.3) are released (excyst) in the intestine. A sporozoite invades an epithelial cell and rounds up to form a trophozoite (BW1.4), which undergoes nuclear division initiating a cycle of asexual multiplication (merogony, schizogony) (BW1.5, 1.6). Merozoites released from asexual stages eventually form sexual stages (male = microgamete, female = macrogamete) (BW1.7, 1.8), which unite to form oocysts.

Unsporulated oocysts are surrounded by a distinct wall and contain a granular cytoplasmic mass within which is indistinct nuclear material (BW1.1, CP10.6). Sporulated oocysts contain four sporocysts, each containing two sporozoites (BW1.2). Some species of *Eimeria* can be speciated by differences in oocyst structure such as size and shape, presence or absence of residuum, polar granules, micropyle, and cap covering the micropyle. The sporozoite is the motile, infectious stage that penetrates the host cell and is identified by its banana shape, single nucleus, refractile (paranuclear) bodies, and PAS-positive granules (BW1.3). The trophozoite is the intracellular, rounded uninucleate stage that develops from the sporozoite or merozoite (BW1.4, CP13.4). Asexual stages referred to as schizonts or meronts develop from sporozoites or merozoites, and immature stages contain from 2 to over 100,000 nuclei (BW1, CP11-14, 16, 17). Each nucleus becomes incorporated into a merozoite, a motile infectious stage structurally similar to the sporozoite (BW1, CP9, 10, 12, 14, 16).

Sexual stages identified as macrogametes (female) are uninucleate and contain peripheral PAS-positive granules (BW1, CP10, 12-15, 17). The immature male stage (microgamont, microgametocyte) is multinucleate (CP15.2, 17.4). When each nucleus becomes incor-

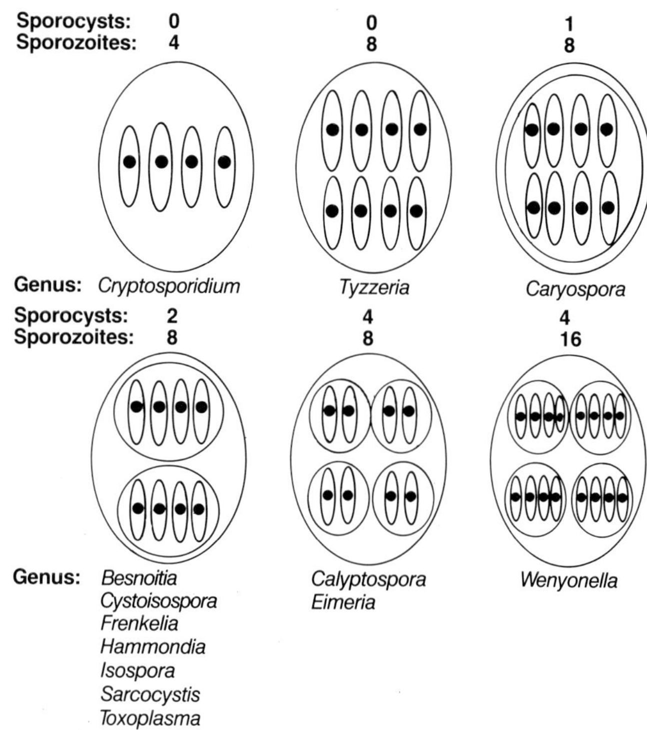

Stylized illustration of sporulated oocysts representative of coccidian genera. Below each oocyst is the name of a genus in which that morphologic form is found. Above each oocyst is the number of sporocysts and sporozoites found in each oocyst of that genus.

porated into a spermlike biflagellate structure (microgamete, BW1.8), the microgamont is mature (CP10.5, 14.3).

The unsporulated oocyst is formed from the macrogamete after it is fertilized by a microgamete (CP10.6, 17.3, 17.6).

Coccidiosis due to *Eimeria* is most common in young animals. Lesions characteristic of *Eimeria* infection are located at the site of parasitism. Destruction of infected cells and surrounding tissue can result in necrosis and hemorrhage (CP9, 10) and in cellular infiltration with architectural change (CP11, 13, 14, 16).

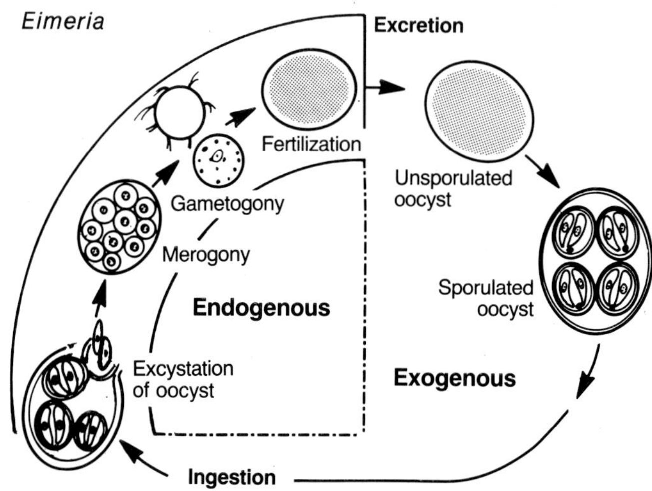

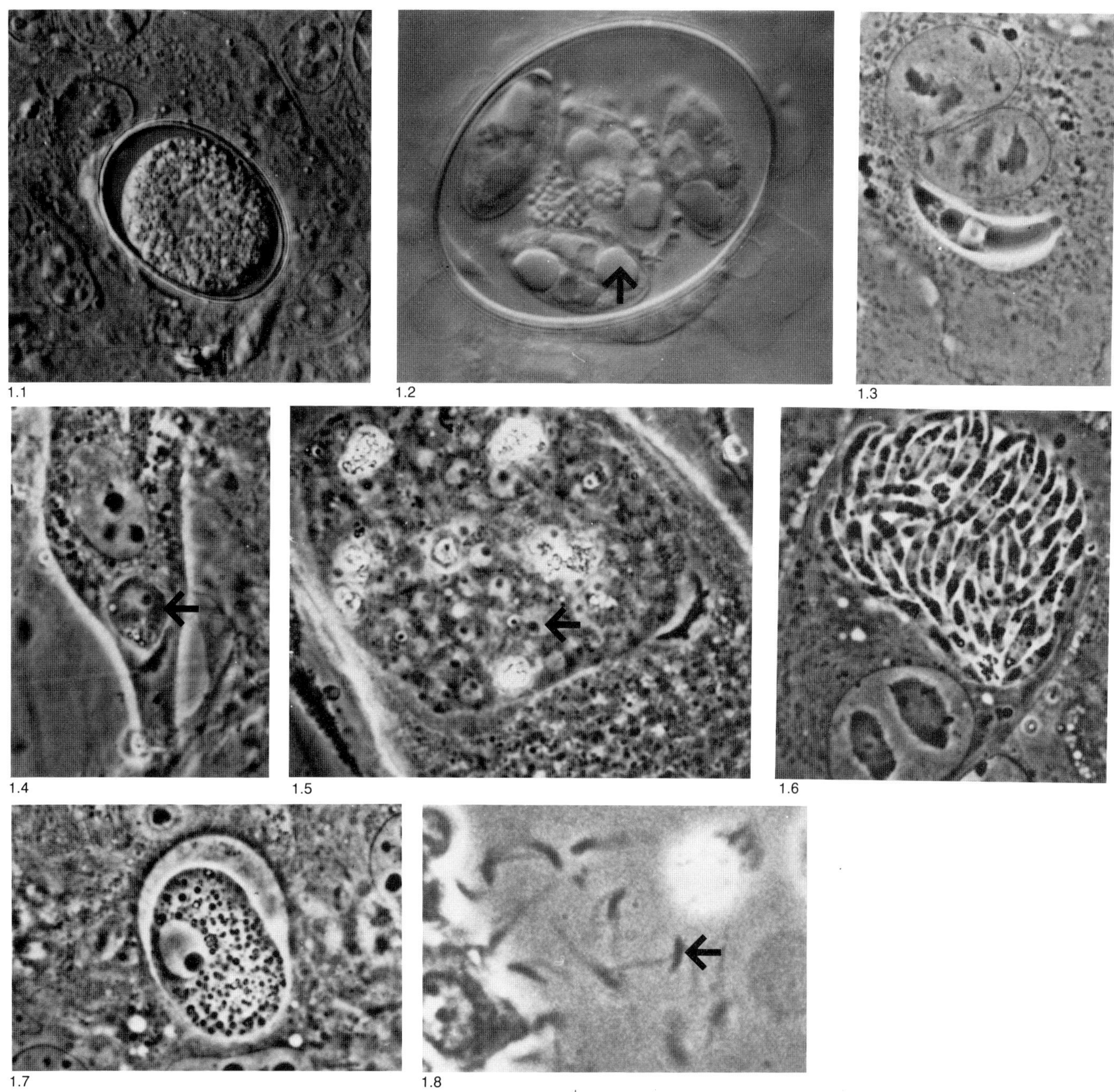

1.1 1.2 1.3
1.4 1.5 1.6
1.7 1.8

Black and white plate 1.—Eimerian life cycle. Stages in mammalian cell culture, live, unstained; either Nomarski interference microscopy (NI) or phase contrast microscopy (PC): 1.1, Unsporulated oocyst of *Eimeria magna* with oocyst wall around granular sporont containing central nuclear area, NI, X 2200.   1.2, Sporulated oocyst of *E. magna* with oocyst wall around granular residuum and four sporocysts, each containing two sporozoites and each sporozoite with central nucleus and distinct posterior refractile body (arrow), NI, X 1700.   1.3, Intracellular sporozoite of *E. larimerensis* adjacent to host cell nucleus surrounded by clear parasitophorous vacuole, PC, X 1200.   1.4, Intracellular trophozoite of *E. zuernii* (arrow) with large nucleus and dark eccentric nucleolus, PC, X 1200.   1.5, Immature meront of *E. zuernii* containing numerous nuclei (arrow), each with distinct nucleolus, PC, X 1600. 1.6, Mature meront of *E. magna* containing numerous merozoites, PC, X 1050.   1.7, Mature macrogamete of *E. magna* in parasitophorous vacuole with numerous granules (wall-forming bodies) throughout cytoplasm and distinct nucleus with dark eccentric nucleolus, PC, X 1100.   1.8, Microgametes of *E. magna* released from microgamont, each microgamete with spindle-shaped body (arrow) and two flagella, PC, X 2200.

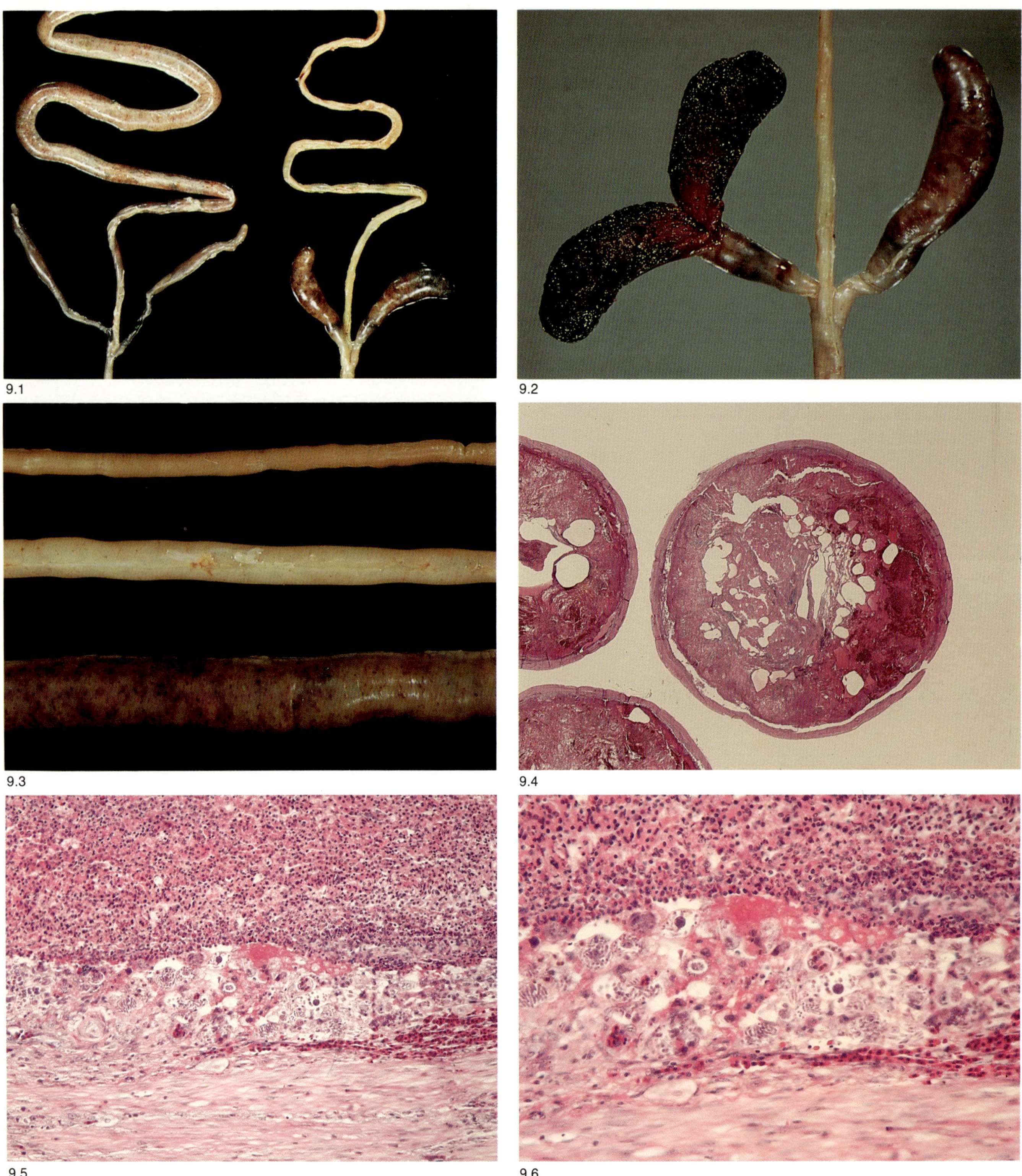

Color plate 9.—*Eimeria* spp. of chickens: 9.1, Digestive tract showing gross lesions of *E. necatrix* in small intestine (left) and *E. tenella* in ceca (right) (84-9379). 9.2, Ceca showing experimental infection with *E. tenella* and necrosis and hemorrhage (84-9380). 9.3, Small intestine containing experimental infection with *Eimeria* and showing *E. necatrix* with distention and multifocal hemorrhage (bottom), *E. acervulina* with moderate edema and no hemorrhage (middle), and uninfected (top) (84-9381). 9.4, Cecum (as in 9.2) showing tissue cross section of *E. tenella* infection resulting in large cecal core with hemorrhage and necrosis, X 5 (84-9382). 9.5, Higher magnification of cecum showing uninfected muscularis (bottom), numerous schizonts of *E. tenella* in submucosa (middle), and necrotic debris (top), X 160 (84-9383). 9.6, Higher magnification of 9.5, X 250 (84-9384).

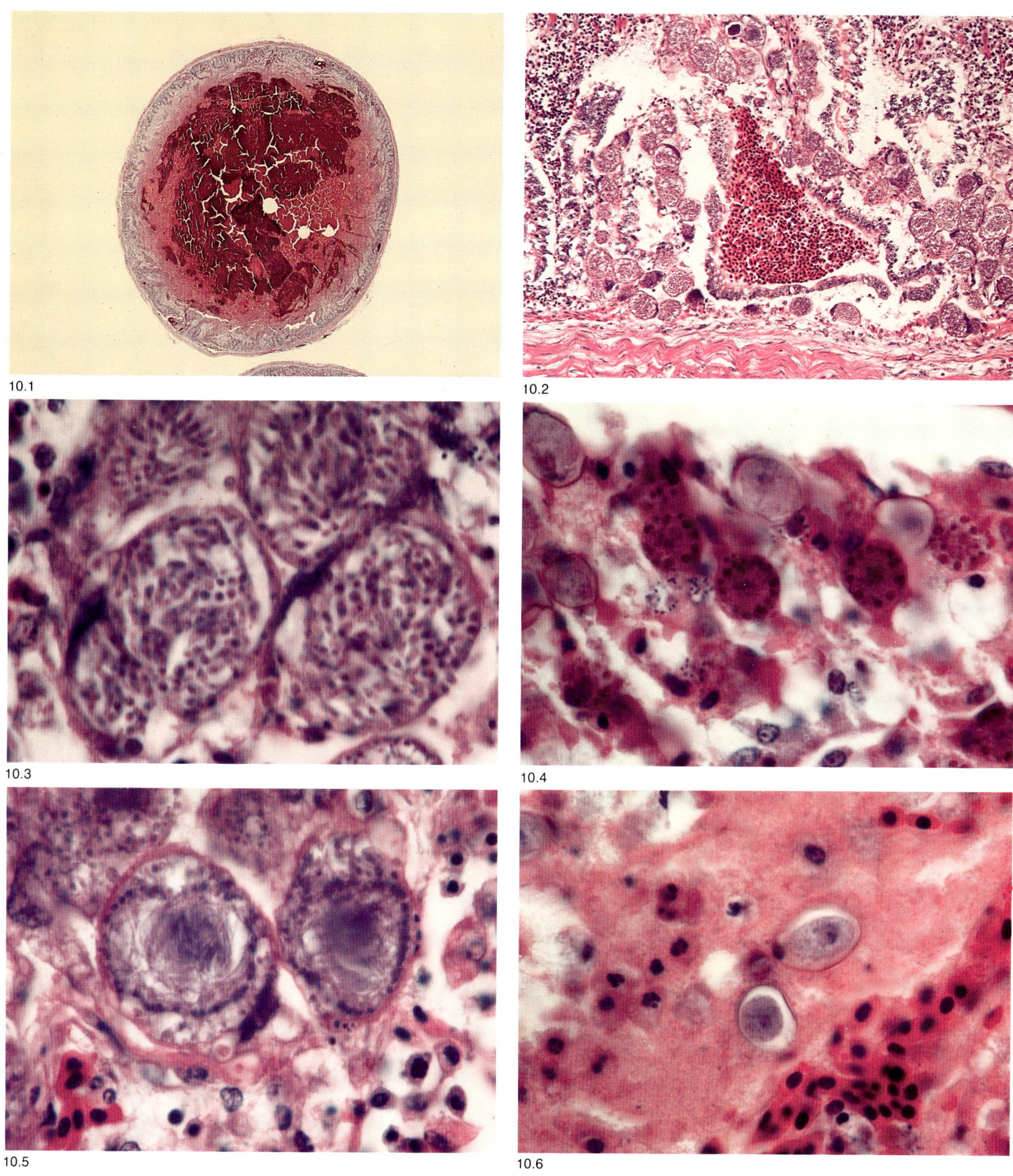

Color plate 10.—*Eimeria necatrix* of chickens: 10.1, Cross section of intestine showing extensive hemorrhage and necrosis, X 7 (84-9385). 10.2, Higher magnification showing numerous schizonts, hemorrhage, and necrosis in submucosa, X 160 (84-9386). 10.3, Mature schizonts containing merozoites, X 1000 (84-9387). 10.4, Macrogametes with eosinophilic peripheral granules, X 1000 (84-9388). 10.5, Microgamonts containing microgametes, X 1000 (84-9389). 10.6, Unsporulated oocysts in lumen, X 1000 (84-9390).

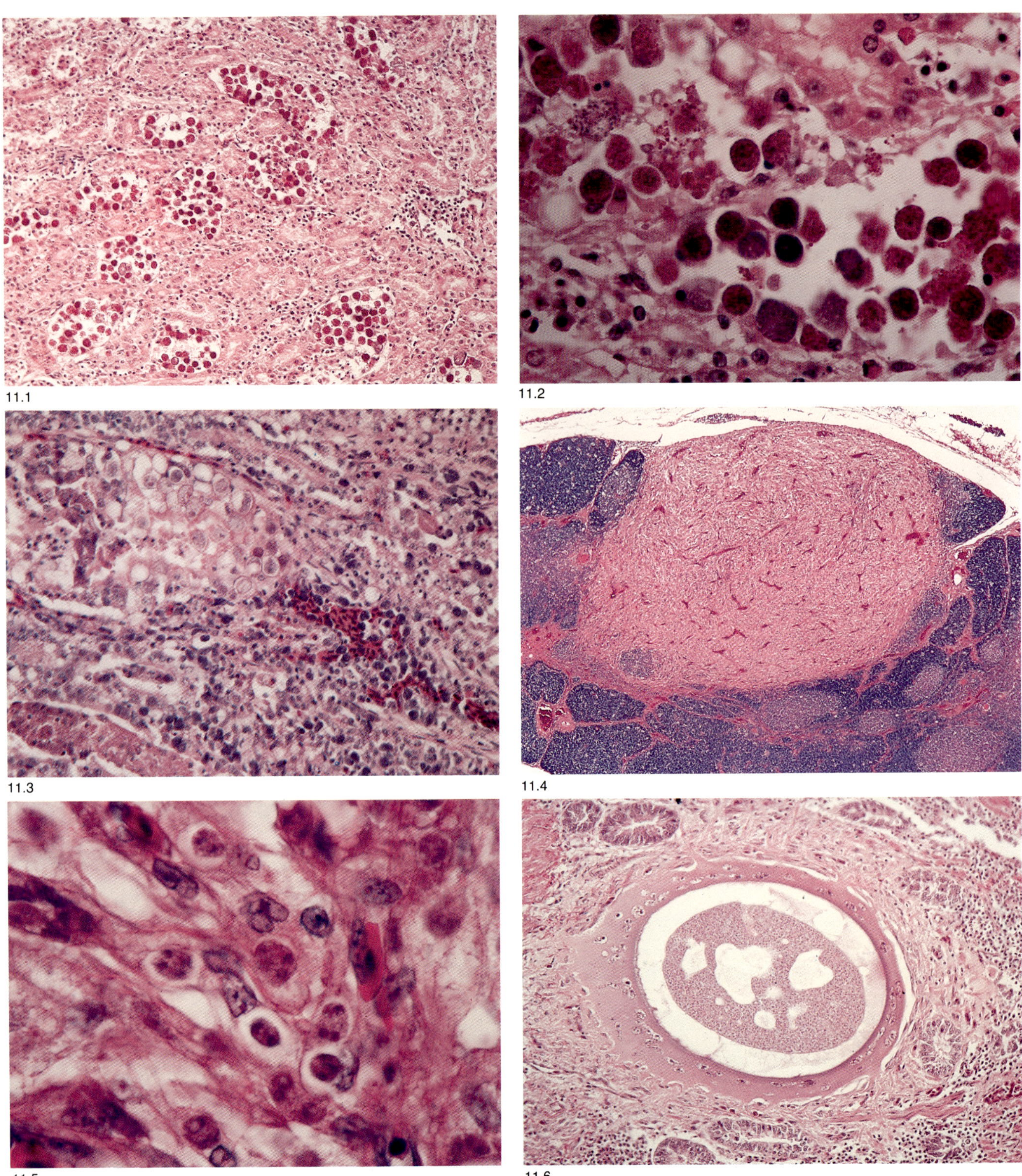

11.1

11.2

11.3

11.4

11.5

11.6

Color plate 11.—*Eimeria* spp. of birds: 11.1, Kidney of goose with gamonts in tubular epithelial cells, X 160 (84-9391).   11.2, Kidney of goose with higher magnification of gamonts, X 630 (84-9395).   11.3, Intestine of whooping crane chick with *E. reichenowi* **oocysts (upper left) and small basophilic** schizonts in macrophages in blood vessels, X 250 (84-5254).   11.4, Pancreas of whooping crane with granuloma containing *E. reichenowi,* X 40 (84-9392).   11.5, Higher magnification of 11.4 showing two to four nucleate schizonts, X 1000 (84-9393).   11.6, Small intestine of swan with large vacuolated schizont of *Eimeria* sp. surrounded by vacuole encapsulated by host tissue, X 160 (84-9394).

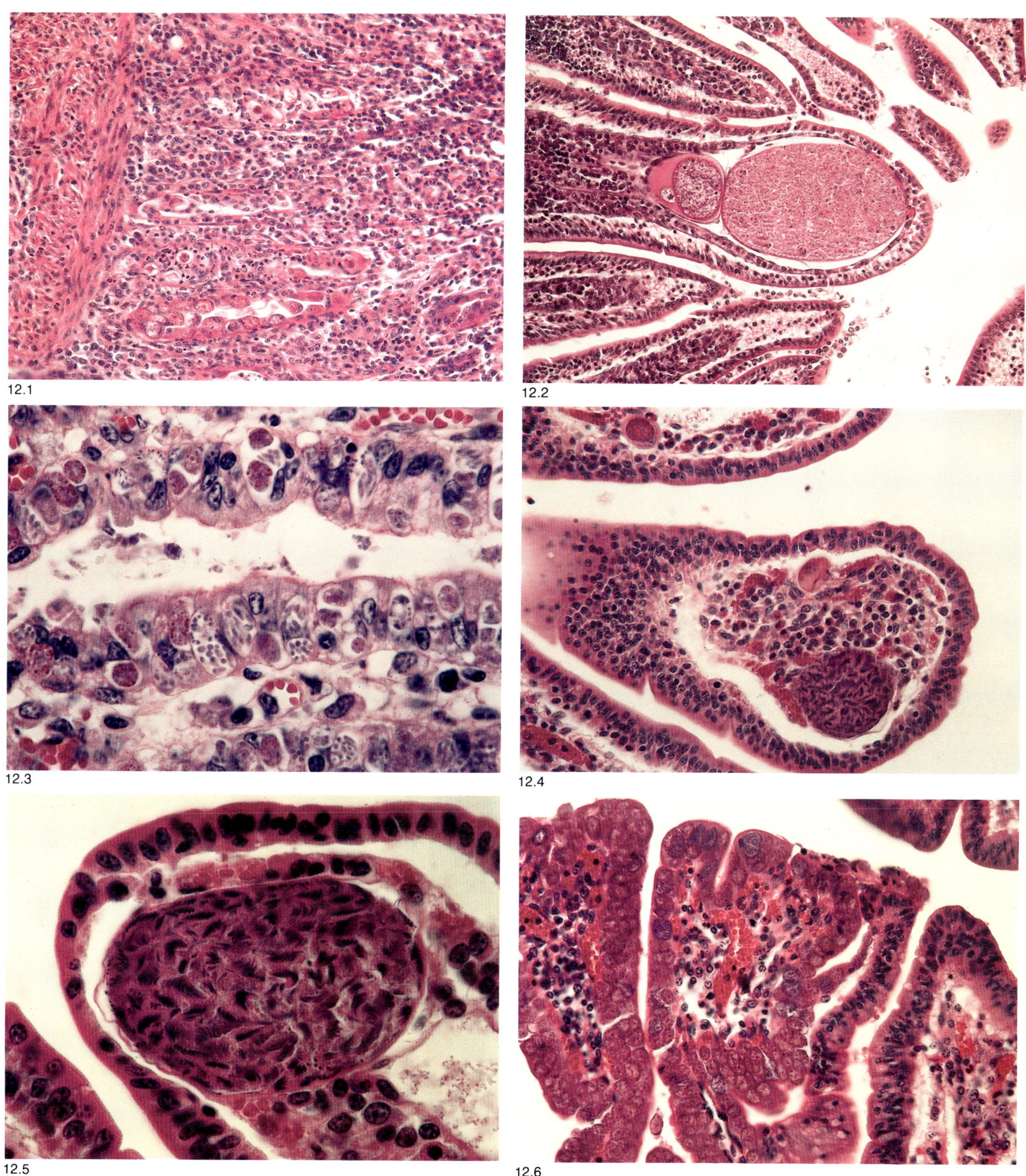

Color plate 12.—*Eimeria* spp. of bovines: 12.1, Small intestine infected with *E. bovis* X 160 (84-9396).   12.2, Villus in small intestine and two schizonts of *E. bovis* containing less mature schizont on left within host cell with hypertrophic nucleus, X 160 (84-9397).   12.3, Epithelium of large intestine with numerous second generation schizonts and gamonts characteristic of *E. zuernii*, X 630 (84-9398).   12.4, Villus in small intestine with oocyst (eosinophilic) and immature microgamont of *E. alabamensis* in lamina propria, X 250 (84-9399).   12.5, High magnification of immature microgamont of *E. alabamensis* showing whirls of dense nuclei, X 630 (84-9400).   12.6, Large intestine with numerous macrogametes of *E. alabamensis*, X 250 (84-9401).

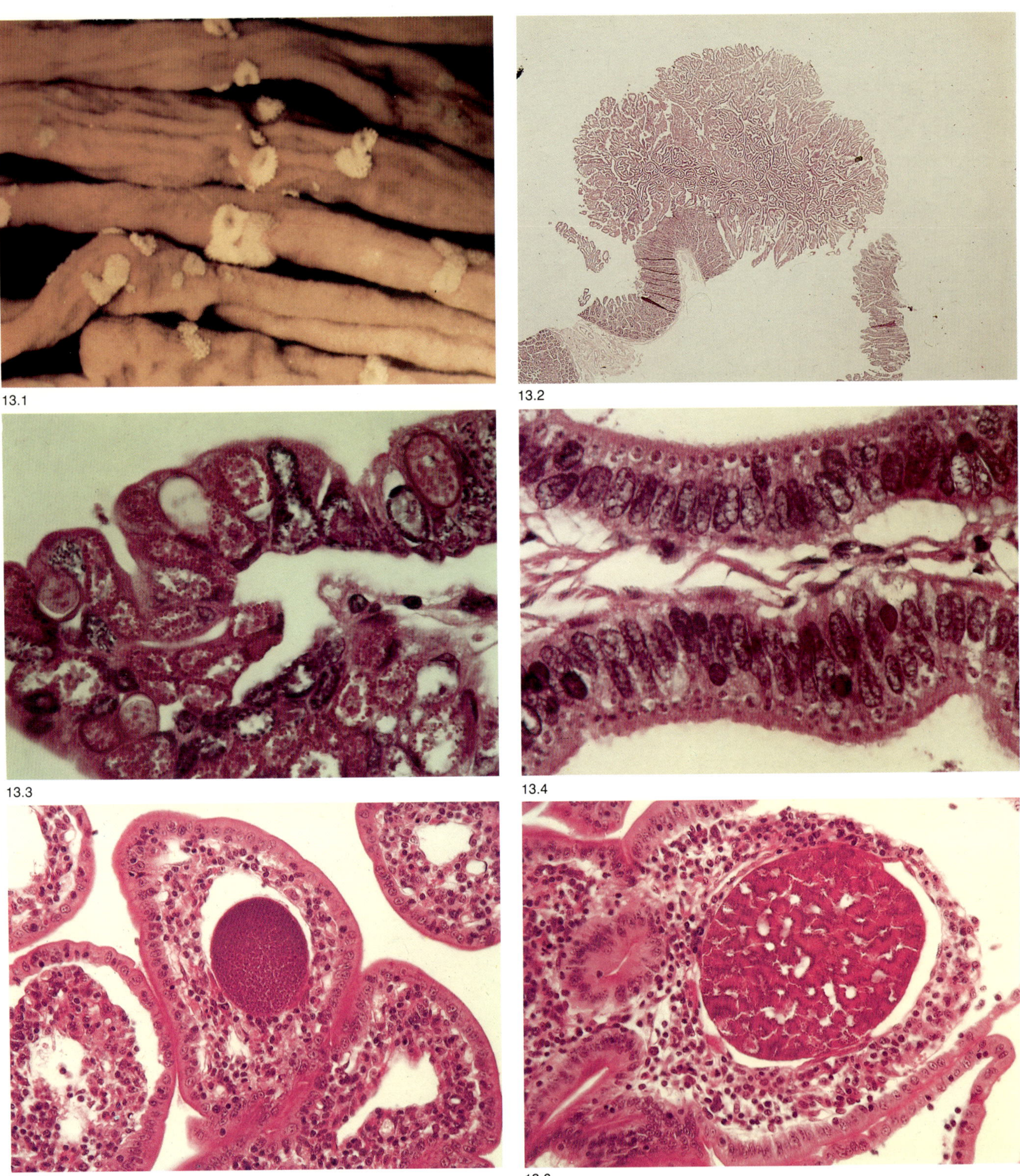

Color plate 13.—*Eimeria* spp. of sheep: 13.1, Large intestine with white polypoid areas of epithelium (oocyst patches) due to *E. ovina* (84-9408).   13.2, Tissue cross section of polyp, X 8 (84-9409).   13.3, Higher magnification of polyp showing numerous eosinophilic macrogametes, basophilic microgamonts, and few oocysts within epithelial cells, X 630 (84-9410).   13.4, Polyp with numerous small meronts between host cell nucleus and brush border, X 630 (84-9411).   13.5, Small intestine with immature schizont of *Eimeria* sp. in lacteal, X 250 (84-9413).   13.6, Small intestine containing large immature schizont of *Eimeria* with compartments formed by infolding of peripheral nuclear layer, X 250 (84-9414).

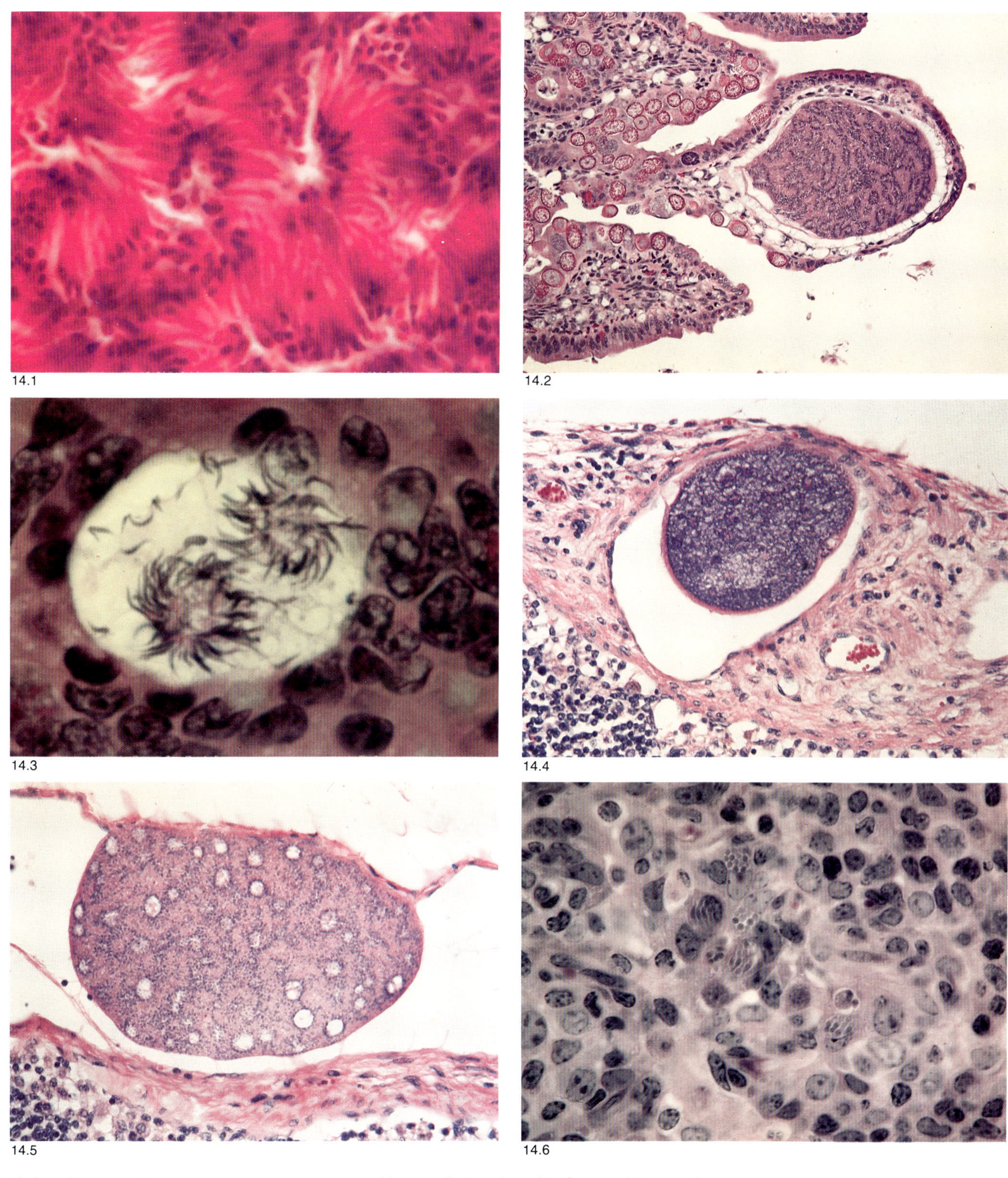

Color plate 14.—*Eimeria* spp. of sheep and goats: 14.1, Small intestine of sheep with whirls of elongate merozoites within mature schizont of *Eimeria* sp., X 1500 (84-9415). 14.2, Large immature schizont in lamina propria of goat with numerous eosinophilic macrogametes and young oocysts in epithelium (species unknown), X 160 (84-9416). 14.3, Intestine of goat with two masses of sperm-like microgametes and free microgametes in host cell vacuole, X 1500 (84-9417). 14.4, Mesenteric lymph node of goat with capsular afferent lymphatic vessel containing large immature schizont of *Eimeria* sp., X 250 (84-9412). 14.5, Mesenteric lymph node of goat with capsular afferent lymphatic vessel containing large schizont of *Eimeria* sp. with nuclei arranged in circular blastophores, X 250 (84-9418). 14.6, Gallbladder of goat with numerous small schizonts of *Eimeria* sp. in lamina propria, X 630 (84-9419).

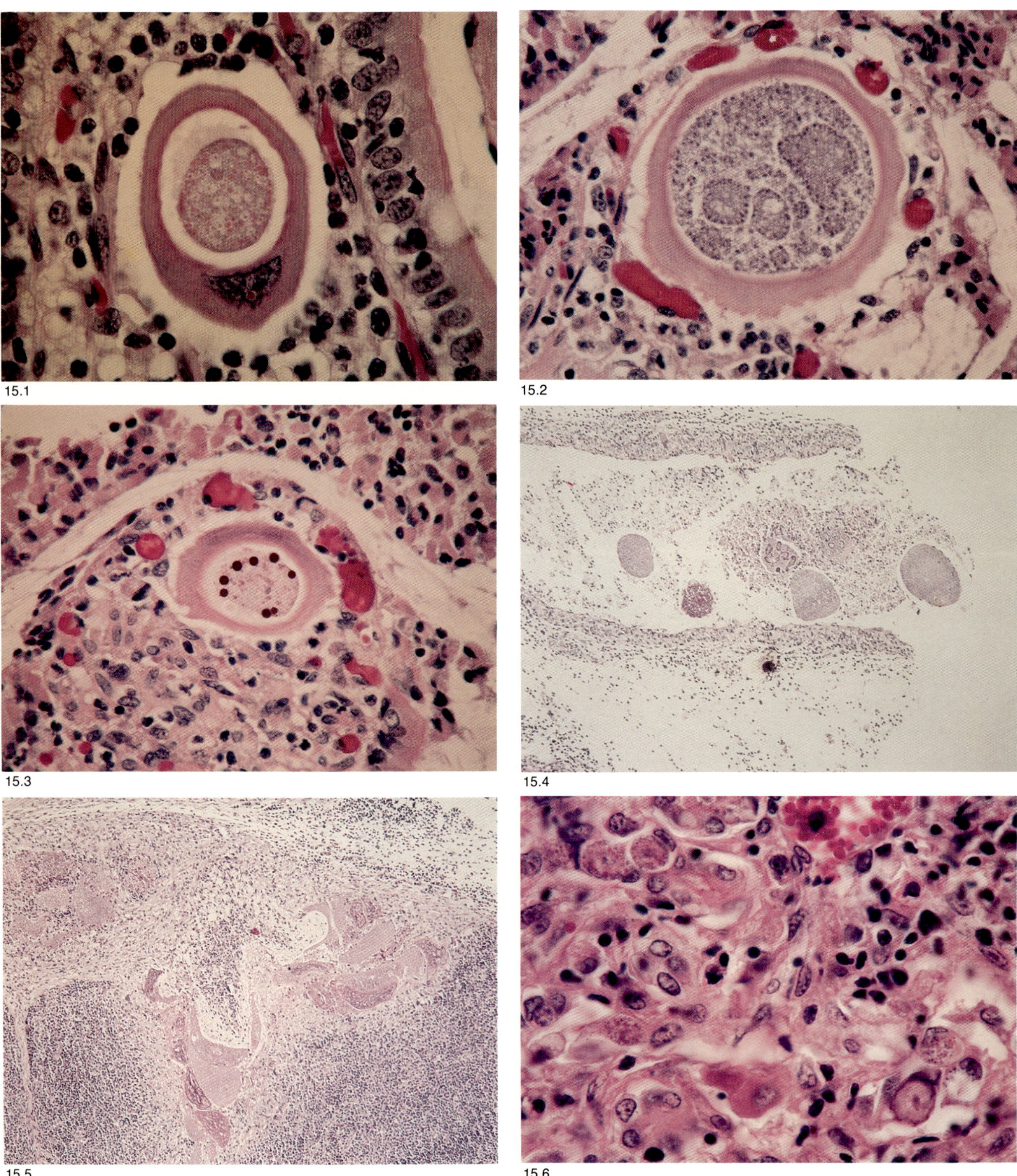

Color plate 15.—*Eimeria* spp. of horses, deer, and goats: 15.1, Small intestine of horse with macrogamont of *E. leuckarti* in lamina propria, X 630 (84-5248).   15.2, Small intestine of horse with microgamont of *E. leuckarti* in lamina propria, X 400 (84-5251).   15.3, Small intestine of horse with developing oocyst in lamina propria, X 400 (84-5250).   15.4, Mesenteric lymph vessel of red deer with numerous large schizonts of *Eimeria* sp., X 60 (84-9402).   15.5, Lymph node of deer with numerous schizonts of *Eimeria*, X 60 (84-9403).   15.6, Liver of goat (*Capra ibex*) with macrogametes containing central nucleus and peripheral granules and with oocysts containing central nucleus and irregular wall of *Eimeria* sp., X 630 (84-9404).

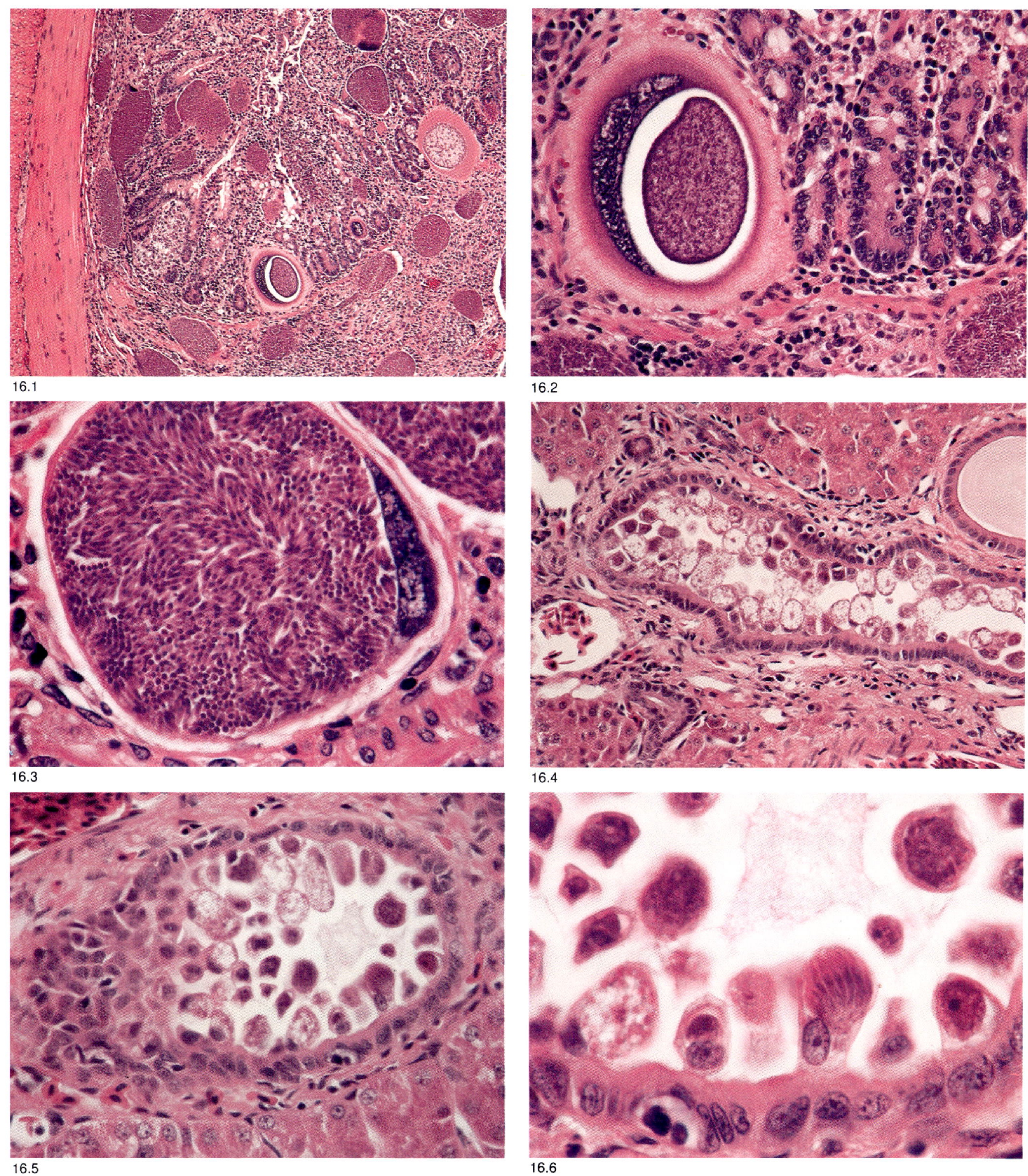

Color plate 16.—*Eimeria* spp. of wallabies and snakes: 16.1, Small intestine of wallaby with numerous large schizonts of *Eimeria* sp., X 60 (84-9405).   16.2, Small intestine of wallaby at higher magnification of schizont of *Eimeria* sp. showing hypertrophied host cell surrounding vacuole containing mature schizont with numerous merozoites, X 250 (84-9406). 16.3, Small intestine of wallaby with hypertrophied host cell nucleus to right of schizont, X 630 (84-9407). 16.4, Bile duct of racer with stages of *Eimeria* sp. in epithelium, X 250 (84-9429). 16.5, Bile duct epithelium of racer with *Eimeria* sp., X 400 (84-9430). 16.6, Bile duct epithelium of racer with schizont (center), macrogamete (far left), and trophozoite (right), X 1000 (84-9431).

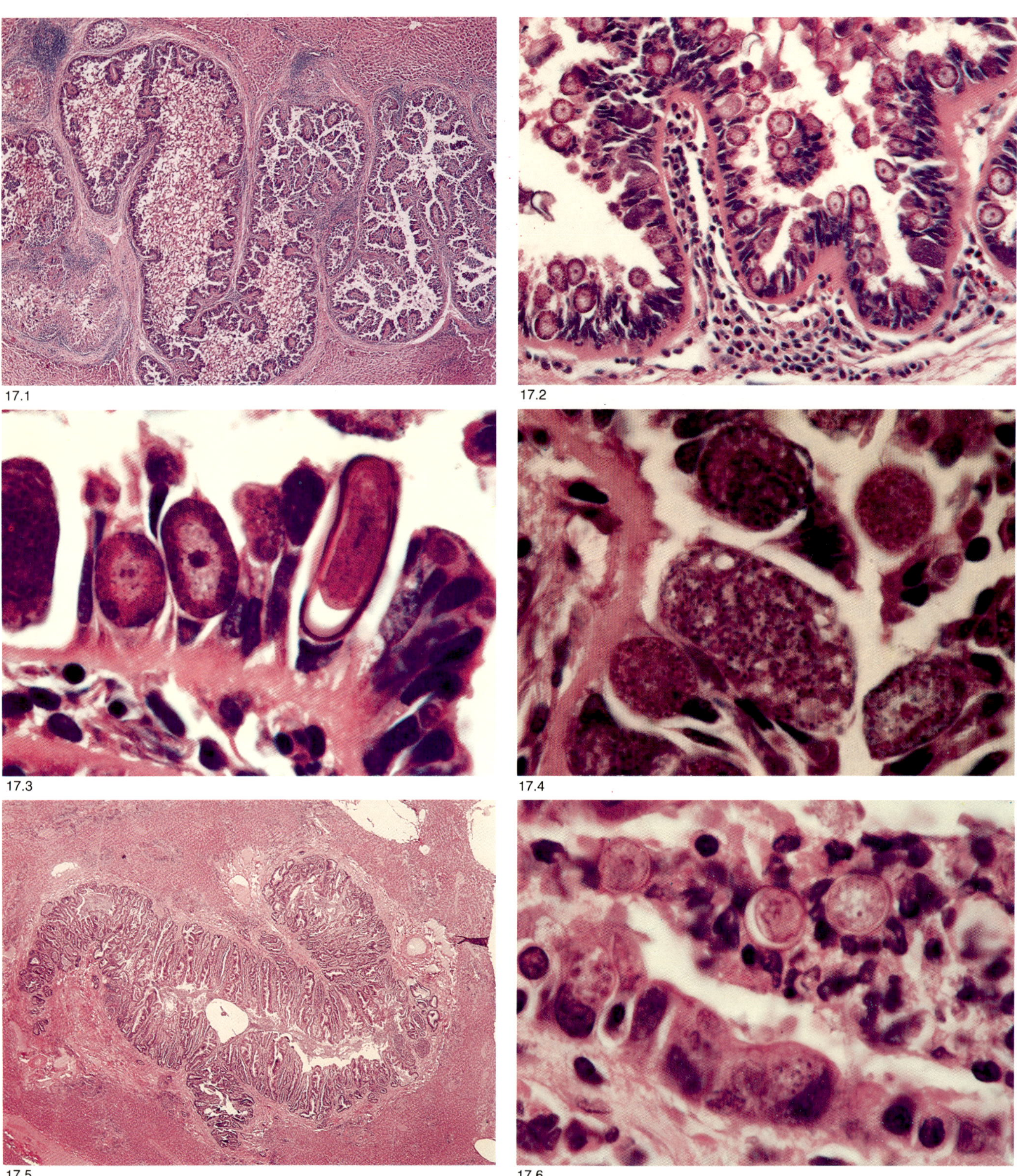

Color plate 17.—*Eimeria* spp. of rabbits and mink: 17.1, Liver of rabbit with grossly dilated bile duct due to *E. stiedae,* X 25 (84-5307). 17.2, Higher magnification of epithelium of bile duct with numerous macrogamonts of *E. stiedae,* X 250 (84-5308). 17.3, Higher magnification of epithelium of bile duct with elongate oocyst (right) and two macrogametes (left), X 1000 (84-9423). 17.4, High magnification of epithelium of bile duct with multinucleate microgamonts of *E. stiedae,* X 1000 (84-5310). 17.5, Liver of mink with grossly dilated bile duct due to *E. hiepei,* X 15 (84-9424). 17.6, Higher magnification of epithelium of bile duct with schizont (bottom left), microgamont (bottom right), and three oocysts surrounded by inflammatory cells (top), X 1000 (84-9425).

Isospora

Isosporan species are coccidian parasites similar in general life cycle and structure to eimerian species but differing most obviously in the oocyst structure (see chart, p. 20). Historically all isoporans were considered to have life cycles identical to those of eimerians, infecting only the digestive tract of a single host species, and were classified as *Isospora* spp. It is now known that certain isosporans can produce encysted asexual stages in extraintestinal tissues of the host, and they have been referred to by some authors as *Cystoisospora* spp.

Isospora spp. are found primarily in carnivores, passeriform birds, amphibians, reptiles, rodents, humans, other primates, and swine (CP18). *Isospora* oocysts found in feces of cattle, sheep, chickens, and turkeys have been accidentally ingested from other hosts.

I. suis of swine illustrates the life cycle and pathogenicity of this genus. Oocysts are unsporulated when shed in feces and sporulate in the environment to become infectious, as do those of *Eimeria.* Following ingestion of sporulated oocysts, sporozoites are released in the intestine, where they parasitize epithelial cells. Sporozoites divide by endodyogeny to form two progenies (CP18.1). After a series of such divisions within the same host cell, merozoites may be released. Merozoites undergo a second type of asexual division (schizogony), in which numerous nuclei develop and many merozoites are formed (CP18.2, 18.3). Following asexual multiplication, merozoites transform into gamonts (CP18.4), which in turn produce oocysts.

Coccidiosis due to *I. suis,* characteristically found in suckling piglets, can be peracute and related to extensive multiplication of asexual stages. Diagnosis of such infections is facilitated by examining mucosal smears for such asexual stages. Oocysts have not yet developed and therefore are not present in the feces. *I. suis* causes villous atrophy, necrotic enteritis, or both. Grossly visible fibrinonecrotic membranes may be found in the small intestine.

The life cycle of certain species of *Isospora* (those referred to as *Cystoisospora*) may involve a transport (paratenic) host. This host becomes infected by ingesting sporulated oocysts and then harbors a monozoic cyst containing a single sporozoite (CP19.3) in various organs. When this host is eaten by the final host, the sporozoite initiates the intestinal cycle (CP19.2, 19.4, 19.5). It is not pathogenic in the transport host but mildly pathogenic in definitive hosts.

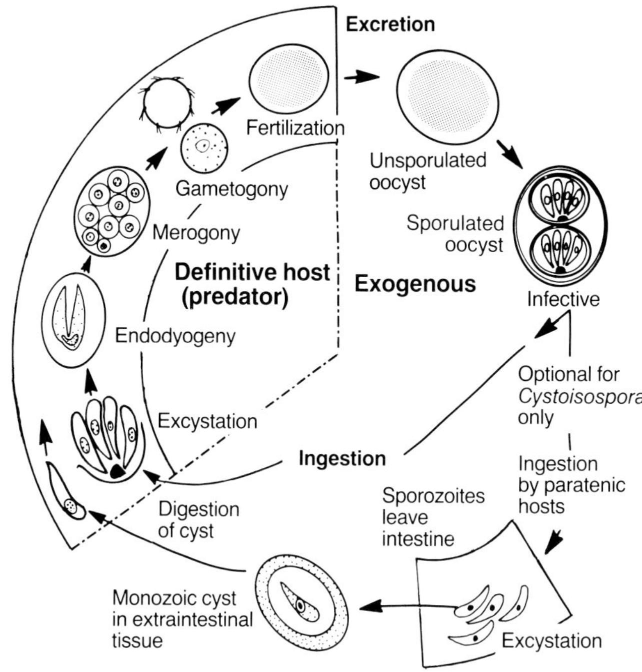

Isospora

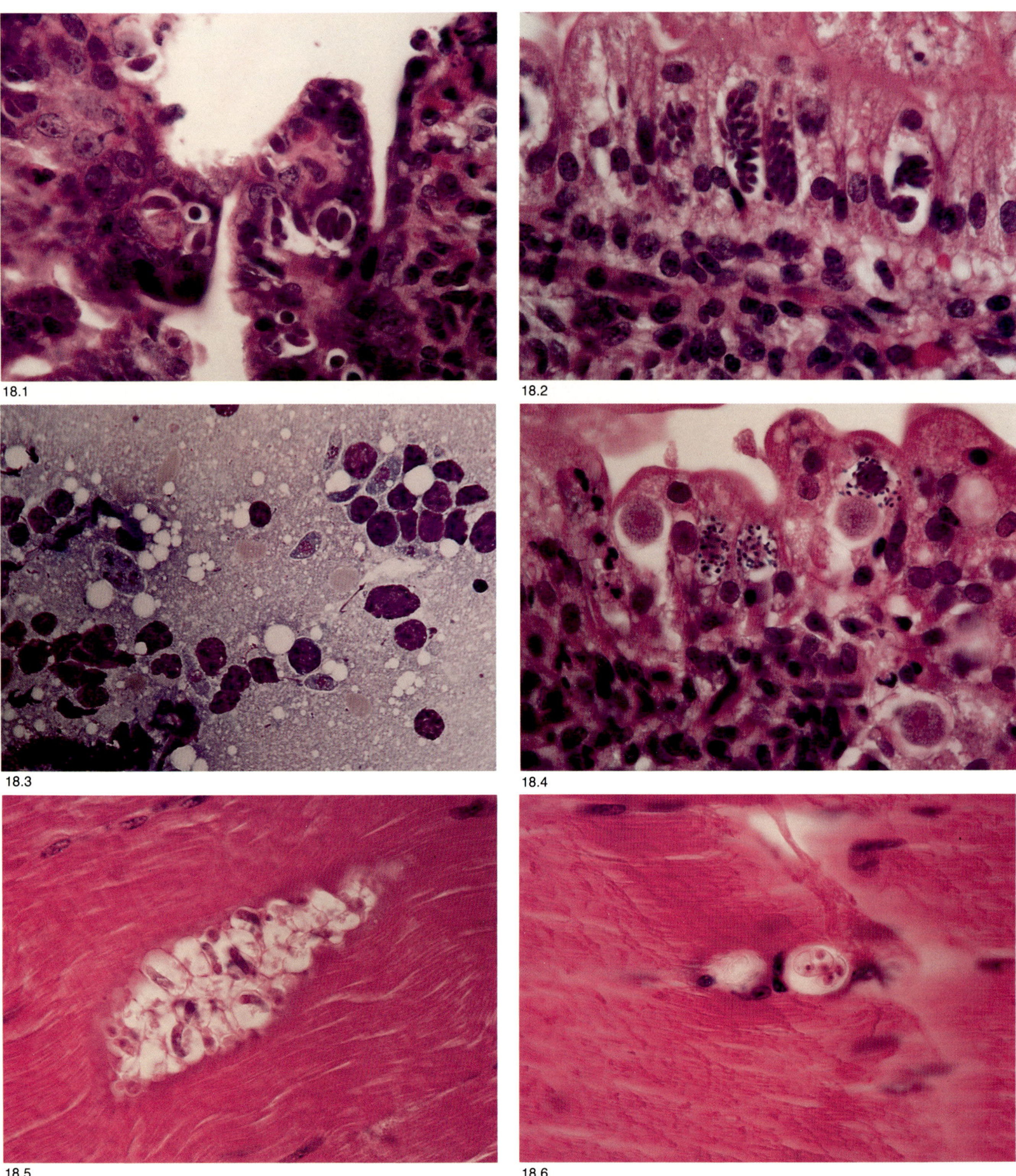

18.1

18.2

18.3

18.4

18.5

18.6

Color plate 18.—*Isospora* spp. of pigs and baboons: 18.1, Small intestine of pig with type I meronts of *I. suis,* X 630 (84-9620). 18.2, Small intestine of pig with type II meronts of *I. suis,* X 630 (84-9619). 18.3, Smear of small intestine of pig with meronts and merozoites of *I.suis,* X 630, Diff-Quik stain (84-9621). 18.4, Small intestine of pig with macrogametes and microgamonts of *I. suis,* X 630 (84-9622). 18.5, Skeletal muscle of baboon with numerous sporulated oocysts of *I. papionis,* X 630 (84-9581). 18.6, Skeletal muscle of baboon with sporulated oocysts of *I. papionis,* X 630 (84-9582).

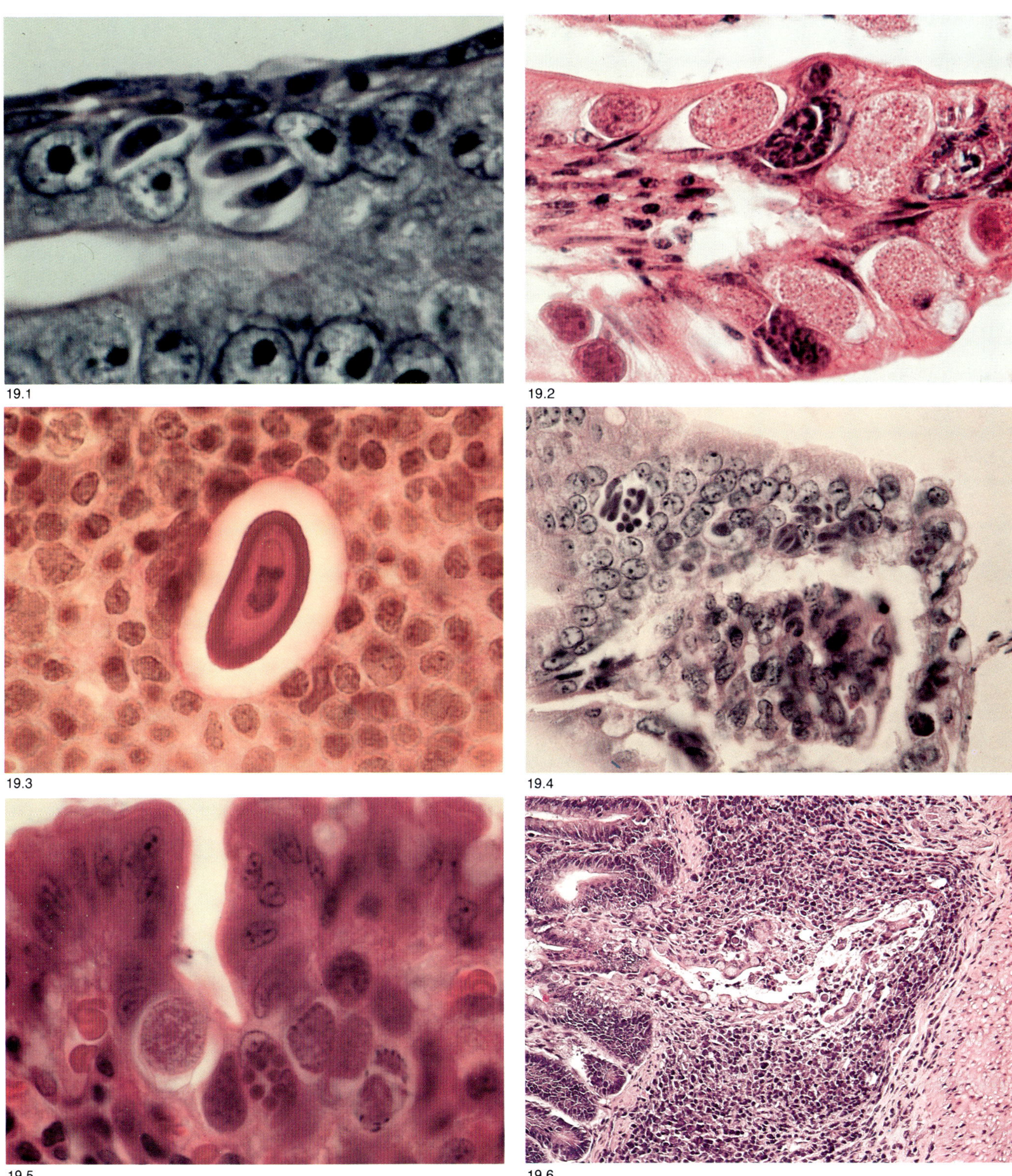

Color plate 19.—*Isospora* spp. and *Cystoisospora* spp. of mammals: 19.1, Small intestine of cat with intraepithelial meronts of *C. rivolta* containing merozoites, X 1500, iron-hematoxylin stain (84-9497).   19.2, Intestine of cat with multinucleate basophilic microgamonts and uninucleate eosinophilic macrogametes of *C. felis* in epithelium, X 1000 (84-9498).   19.3, Mesenteric lymph node of mouse with smear of monozoic cyst of *C. felis* showing clear white space surrounding thick darkly stained wall enclosing single sporozoite, X 1500, PAS stain (84-9499).   19.4, Small intestine of dog with several mature meronts of *C. ohioensis* in epithelium, X 630 (84-9500).   19.5, Small intestine of dog with various asexual and sexual stages of *I. neorivolta,* X 1000 (84-9501).   19.6, Small intestine of dog with developmental stages of *Isospora* sp. extending into submucosa, X 160 (84-9502).

Caryospora

Coccidia of the genus *Caryospora* are found primarily in birds and snakes. Members of the genus were once thought to infect a single host species. Recent studies show that species of *Caryospora* have two-host life cycles, in which the hosts have a predator-prey relationship. There are owl-mouse and snake-mouse cycles. Unsporulated oocysts are shed in the feces of the predatory or definitive host (birds and reptiles). Sporulated oocysts contain a single sporocyst with eight sporozoites. Ingestion of sporulated oocysts by the definitive host results in merogony, gamogony, fertilization, and formation of oocysts in the intestinal epithelium (CP20.1, 20.2). Ingestion of sporulated oocysts by the prey or intermediate host (rodents) results in extraintestinal merogony, gamogony, fertilization, sporulation, and formation of a caryocyst typically containing a single sporozoite in the tongue, dermis, and hypodermis (CP20.3, 20.6). Ingestion of the prey whose tissues contain caryocysts results in merogony (two generations), gamogony, and oocyst formation in the intestine of the predator.

Little is known of the pathogenicity of *Caryospora*. Experimentally infected mice develop facial edema and some die. Clinical illness has not been reported for definitive hosts.

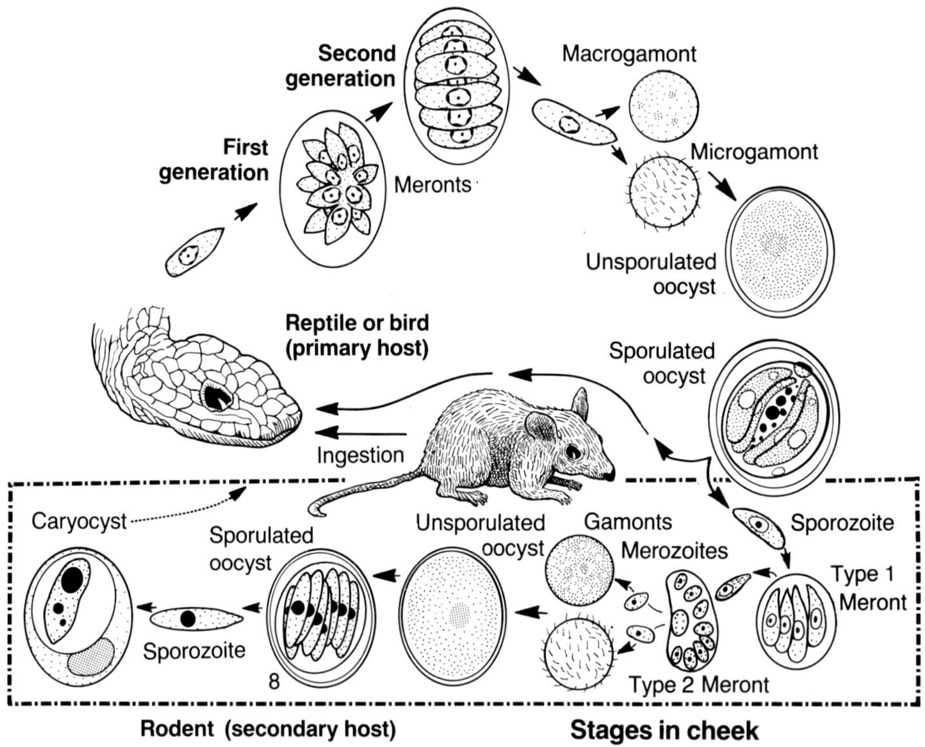

Caryospora

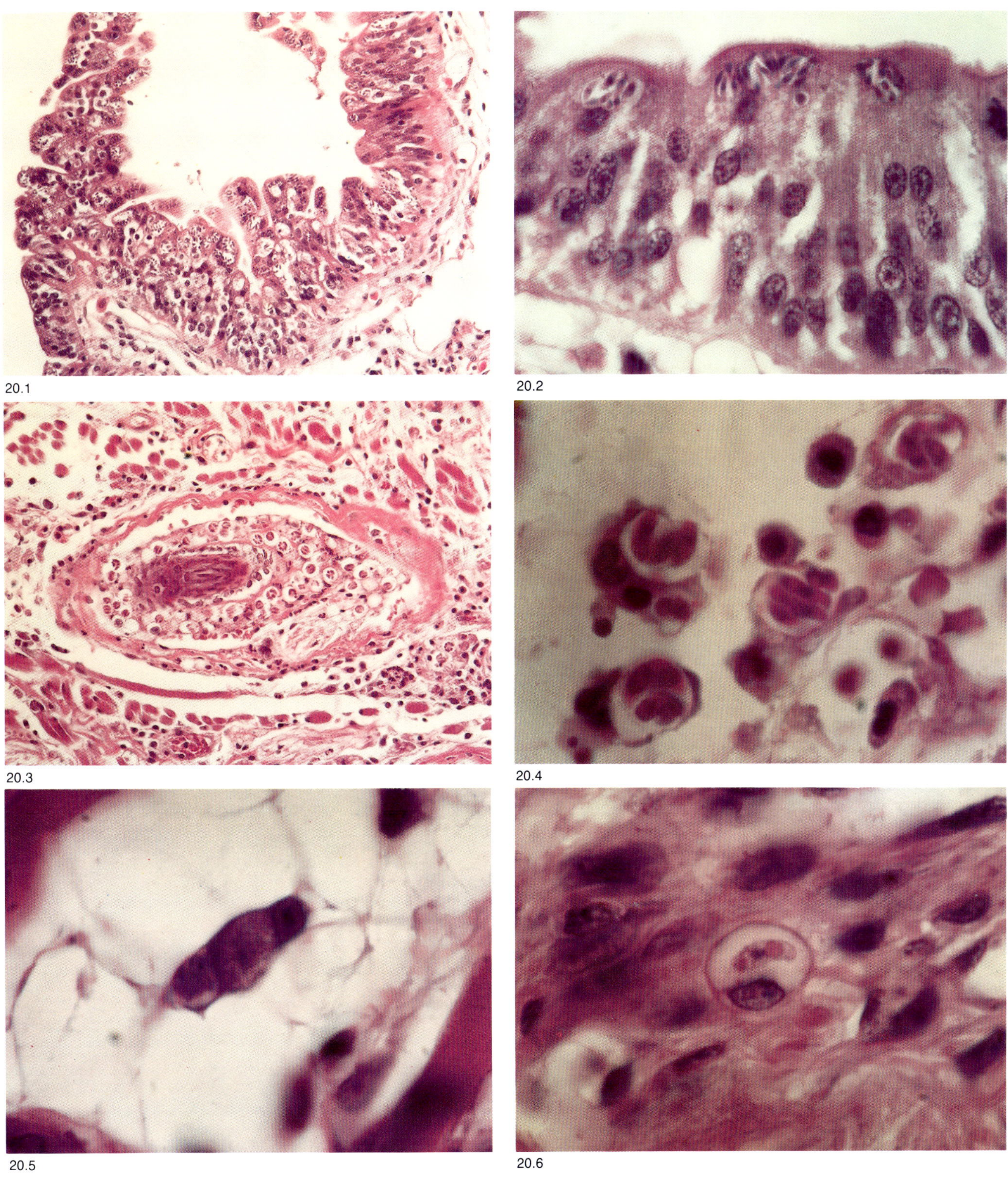

Color plate 20.—*Caryospora bigenetica* of snakes and mice: 20.1, Small intestine of rattlesnake with numerous schizonts in epithelium, X 250 (84-9516). 20.2, Higher magnification of rattlesnake intestine with schizonts, X 1000 (84-9517). 20.3, Skin of mouse with numerous sporulated oocysts within clear vacuoles of host cells surrounding densely stained hair shaft, X 250 (84-9518). 20.4, Skin of mouse with sporulated oocysts containing sporozoites, X 1500 (84-9519). 20.5, Tongue of mouse containing microgametocyte (left) and macrogamete (middle) in host cell with nucleus on right, X 1500 (84-9520). 20.6, Tongue of mouse with caryocyst containing single sporozoite within host cell in lamina propria, X 1500 (84-9521).

Cryptosporidium

Coccidia of the genus *Cryptosporidium* are found in mammals, birds, fish, and reptiles. Historically, numerous species of *Cryptosporidium* were each thought to infect a single host species, but recent studies show that an isolate of *Cryptosporidium* from one mammalian host can infect several other mammalian host species. Transmission is direct. Unusually small (ca. 5 μm) sporulated or unsporulated oocysts are shed in the feces (CP22). On ingestion or inhalation of sporulated oocysts, sporozoites are released and infect the epithelium in the digestive or respiratory tract. Although asexual and sexual stages of *Cryptosporidium* are morphologically similar to those of other coccidia, they possess some unique distinguishing characteristics. All stages are small (ca. 1-6 μm in diameter) and are located at the microvillar surface of epithelial cells (BW2). When viewed with light microscopy, these stages appear as dots (CP21). Meronts contain only four to eight merozoites. Some oocysts sporulate in situ and contain four sporozoites.

Cryptosporidium is typically found in neonatal or young animals. Disease is not always present. *Cryptosporidium*, however, has been associated with clinical enteritis (CP21.3) in several hosts, including man and domestic animals, and with respiratory illness in man and domestic birds.

Diagnosis has been recently facilitated by identifying oocysts in the feces with phase-contrast microscopy and several staining procedures formerly used for acid-fast bacteria.

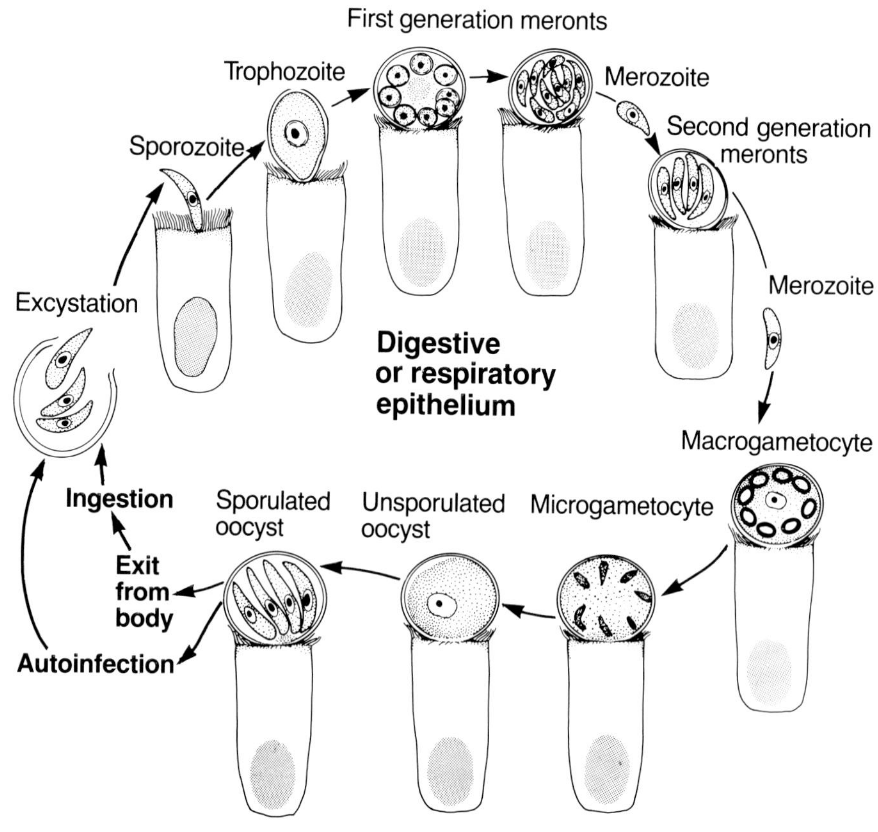

Cryptosporidium

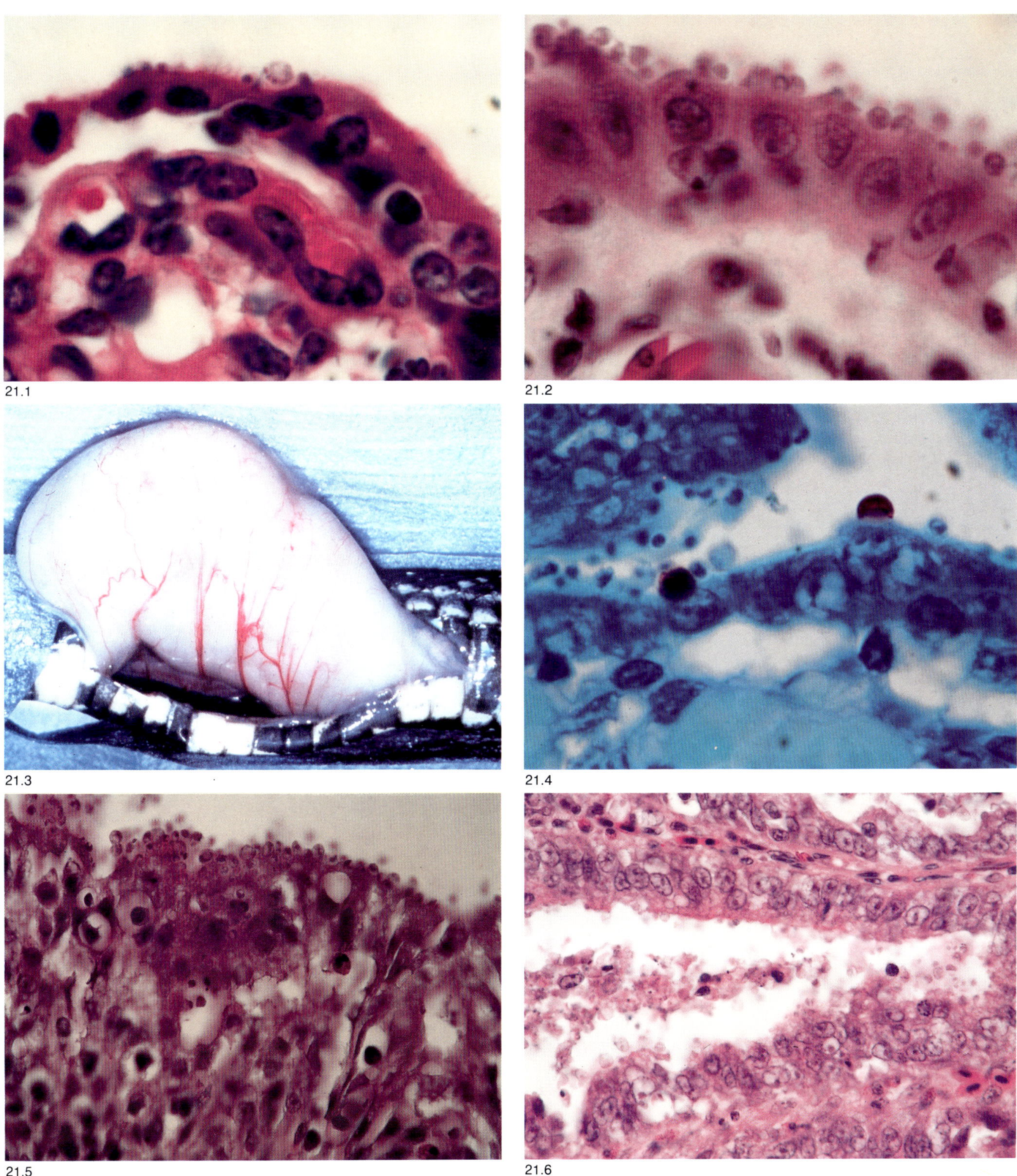

21.1

21.2

21.3

21.4

21.5

21.6

Color plate 21.—*Cryptosporidium* spp. of animals: 21.1, Small intestine of calf with organisms within surface of epithelium and small densely stained stages (left) and larger oocyst (right), X 1500 (84-9433).   21.2, Stomach of snake with numerous stages within gastric epithelium, X 1500 (84-9434). 21.3, Hypertrophied stomach of black rat snake with cryptosporidiosis.   21.4, Small intestine of calf containing two red oocysts and numerous developing stages within epithelium with acid-fast stain demonstrating positivity of mature oocysts but not of other stages, X 1500 (84-9435). 21.5, Tracheal epithelium of turkey with numerous stages, X 630 (84-9436).   21.6, Kidney tubules of finch with numerous stages within lumen and in tubular epithelial cells, X 630 (84-9437).

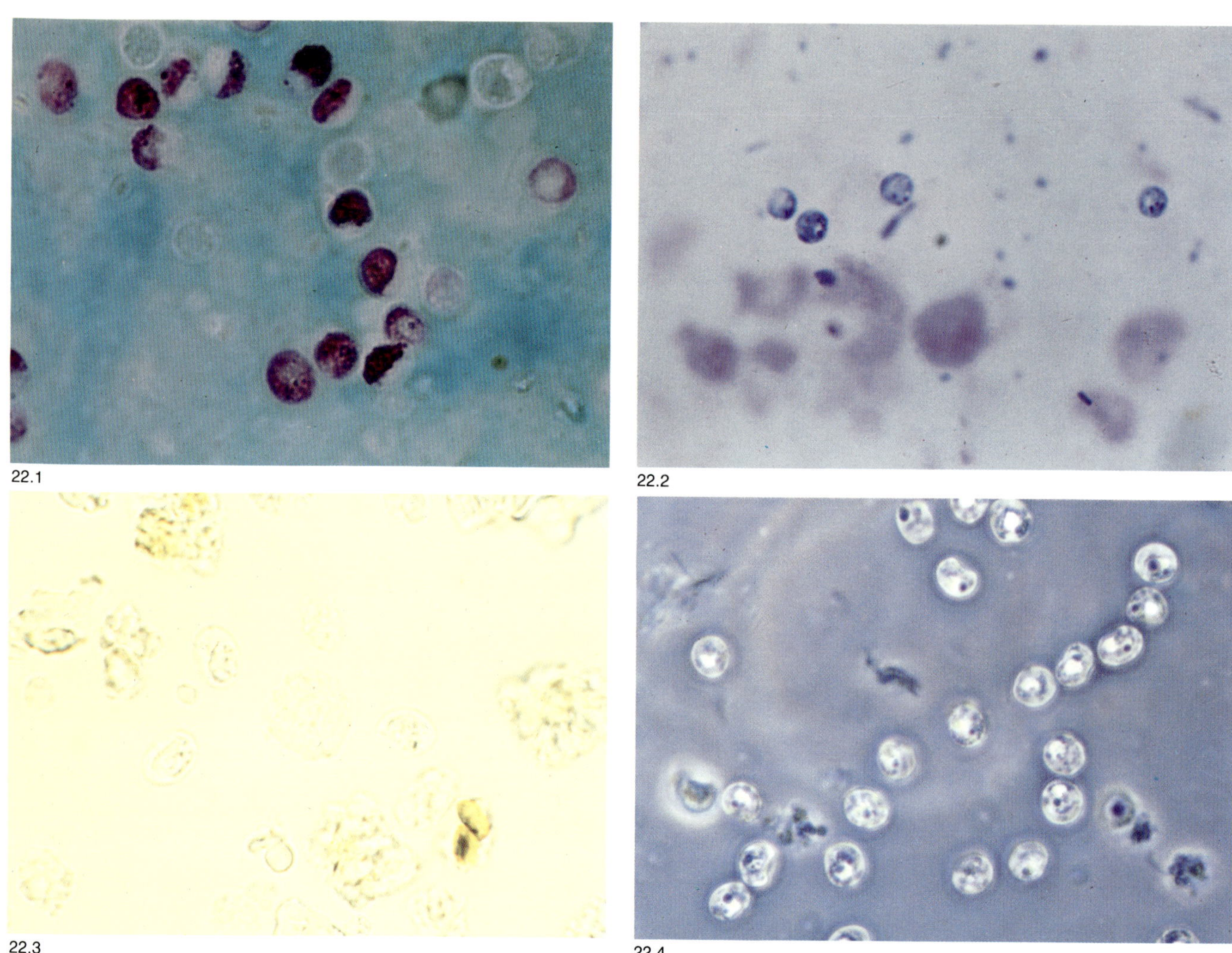

22.1

22.2

22.3

22.4

Color plate 22.—*Cryptosporidium* spp. of calves: 22.1, Fecal smear with oocysts stained red and yeasts green, X 1500, acid-fast stain (84-9432).   22.2, Fecal smear with oocysts stained blue, X 750, Giemsa stain. 22.3, Fecal float with unstained oocysts suspended in water and viewed with bright field microscopy, X 1500.   22.4, Fecal float with unstained oocysts suspended in sugar solution and viewed with phase-contrast microscopy, X 1500.

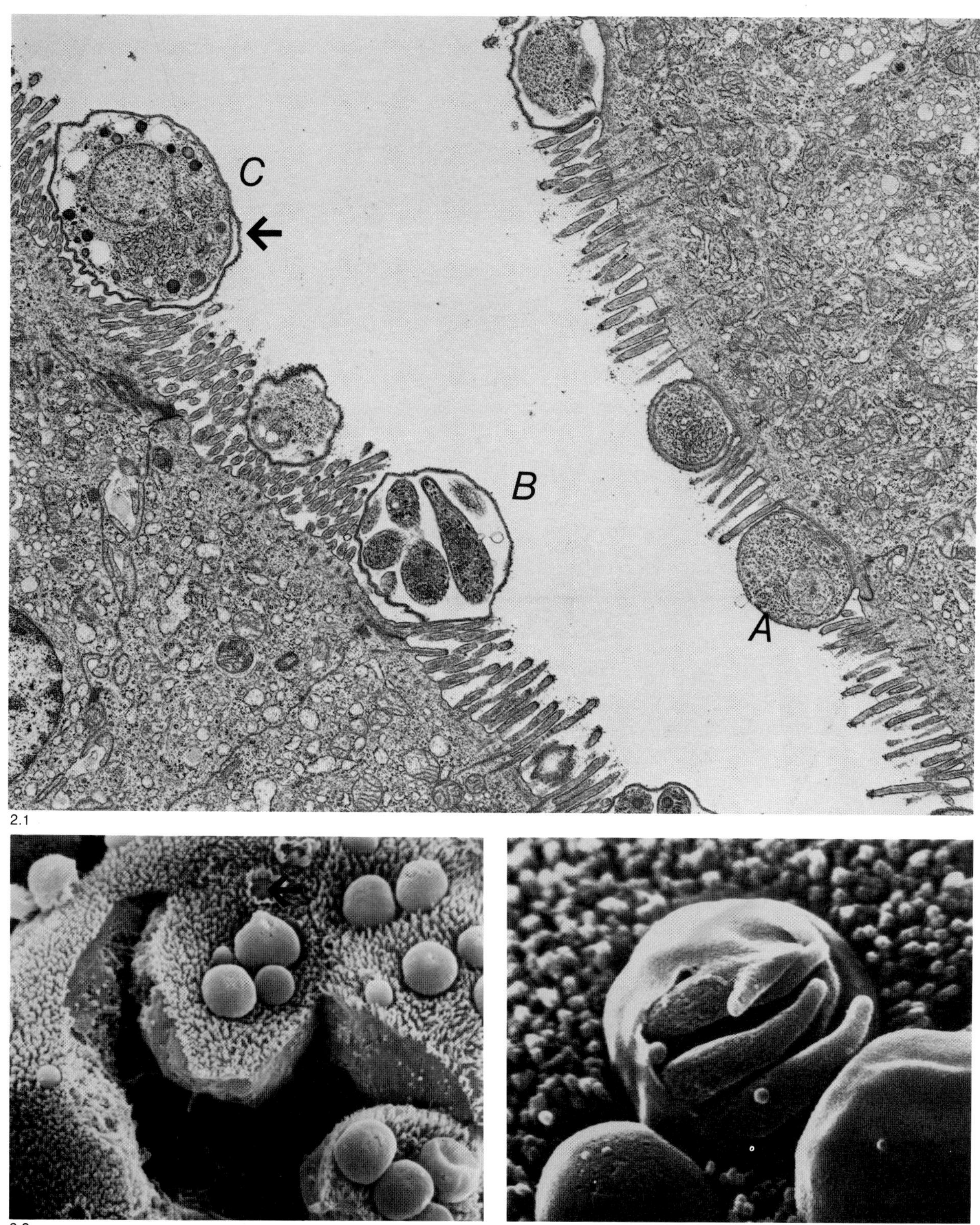

Black and white plate 2.—Electron micrographs of *Cryptosporidium* sp. of sheep. Stages in epithelium of small intestine of week-old lamb: 2.1, Trophozoite (*A*), meront (*B*), and macrogamete-like stage (*C*) among microvilli at surface of epithelial cells, each stage intracellular and surrounded by host cell membrane (arrow), transmission electron microscopy, X 5720. 2.2, Numerous cryptosporidia on surface of epithelial cells with craterlike area (arrow) remaining where organism has been detached, scanning electron microscopy, X 3500. 2.3, Meront with outer membrane missing, exposing merozoites within, scanning electron microscopy, X 18,000.

Sarcocystis

Sarcocystis is a genus of cyst-forming coccidia with an obligatory two-host life cycle. Cysts are found primarily in muscles of wild and domestic herbivores. Carnivores that prey on herbivore hosts become infected and serve as definitive hosts when zoites released by digestion of mature cysts invade the intestinal epithelium and develop directly into gamonts. Fertilization is followed by formation of oocysts, which sporulate within the intestine (CP23.1, 23.2) and are shed as infective oocysts or sporocysts (CP23.3) in the feces of the carnivore. On ingestion of oocysts or sporocysts by susceptible herbivorous mammals or birds, sporozoites are released (excyst) in the intestine. They migrate to arterial vessels, where they develop into meronts (CP23.4, 25.1). Merozoites liberated from these meronts initiate a second generation of meronts in capillaries throughout the body (CP23.5, BW3). Merozoites liberated from second generation meronts enter mononucleate cells found in the circulation and undergo endodyogeny within the cytoplasm of these cells (CP23.6). Merozoites from the circulation enter the heart and skeletal muscle cells and the neural tissue, where they develop into immature noninfective sarcocysts that contain unicellular metrocytes (CP24.4). Metrocytes produce bradyzoites that are infective for the predator animal and whose presence characterizes a mature sarcocyst (CP24.5, 24.6, 25.3-25.6). Sarcocysts of some species remain microscopic (CP24.5, 24.6), whereas others become visible to the unaided eye (CP26.5, 26.6).

Some species of *Sarcocystis* are pathogenic to the herbivore intermediate host. Acute lesions characterized by hemorrhage, edema, and necrosis are associated with the maturation of second generation meronts. Macroscopic lesions observed postmortem may include generalized serous atrophy of fat, excessive yellowish fluid in all body cavities, watery blood, petechial hemorrhage in the heart and pericardium, serosa of the gastrointestinal tract and urinary bladder, edema and hemorrhage of lymph nodes, and alternate pale and dark striping or mottling of skeletal muscles. Microscopically, hemorrhage may be seen in all organs, and mononuclear cell infiltration into the perivascular and intestinal tissues of the heart, skeletal muscles, lung, liver, and kidney may be mild to severe (CP24.1-24.3). Regenerative changes are most often associated with the myocardium. Chronic lesions characterized by muscle atrophy and myositis are associated with mature sarcocysts. Specific macroscopic lesions may not always be seen postmortem. Microscopic lesions may include myositis and myocarditis. Most definitive hosts are clinically unaffected by *Sarcocystis* infection.

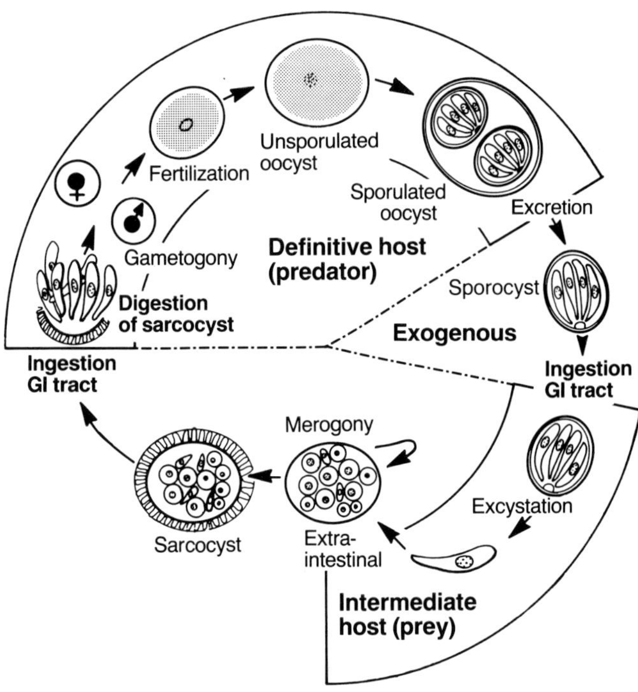

Sarcocystis

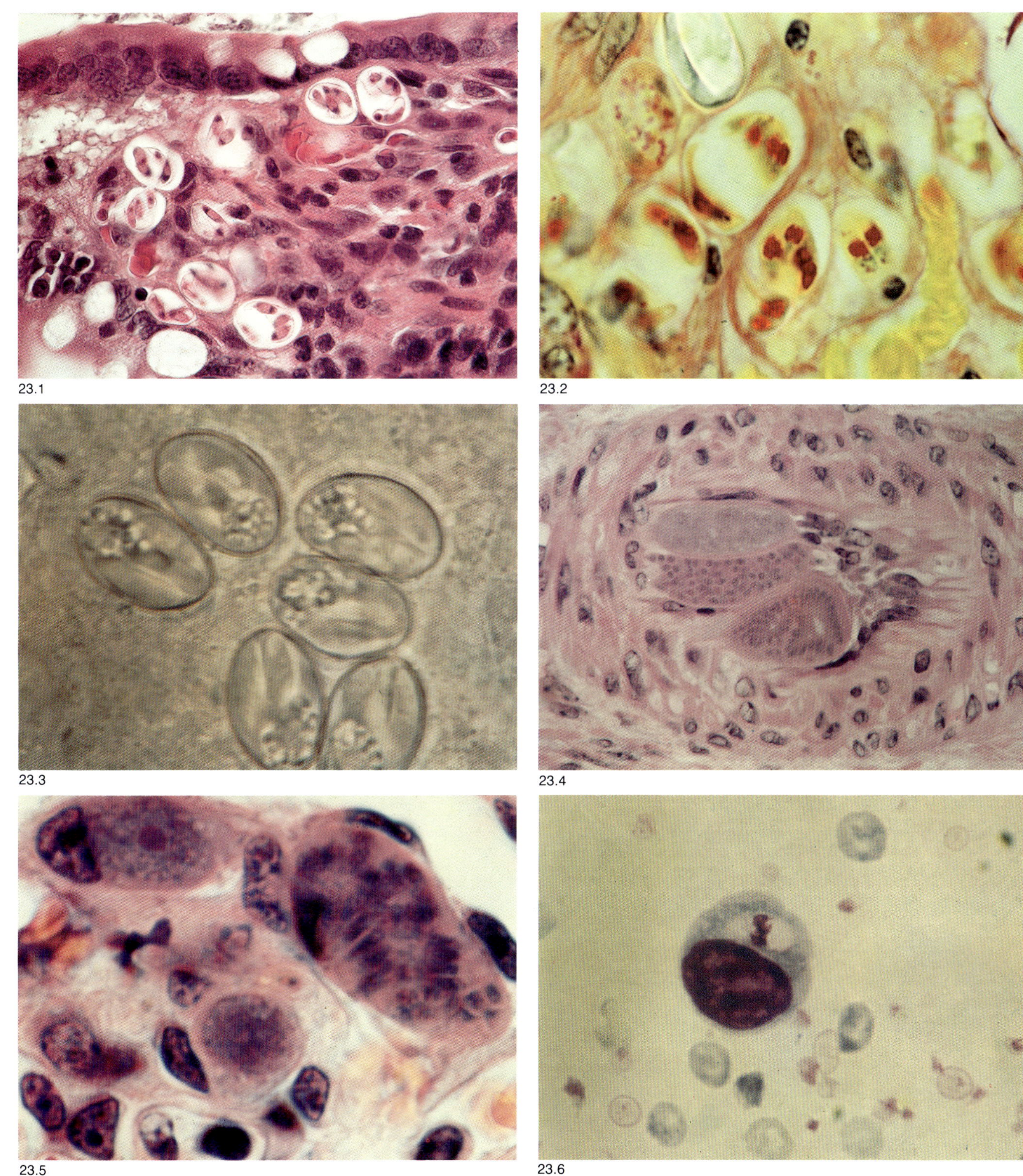

23.1

23.2

23.3

23.4

23.5

23.6

Color plate 23.—*Sarcocystis cruzi* (syn., *S. bovicanis*) of canines and bovines: 23.1, Small intestine of dog with numerous sporulated oocysts in subepithelium, X 630 (84-9503). 23.2, Small intestine of dog with sporulated oocysts containing sporozoites with yellow cytoplasm and red polysaccharide and green nucleoplasm, X 1000, Whipf's polychrome stain (84-9504). 23.3, Feces of dog containing sporocysts of *S. cruzi,* each with four sporozoites and granular residuum, X 1500, unstained (84-9505). 23.4, Renal artery of calf containing three developing meronts, each with numerous nuclei occluding lumen of vessel, X 630 (84-9515). 23.5, Renal glomerulus of calf containing three intravascular meronts, two immature (left) and one mature with merozoites (right), X 1500 (84-9507). 23.6, Peripheral blood smear of calf with mononucleate host cell containing binucleate merozoite, X 1500, Giemsa stain (84-9508).

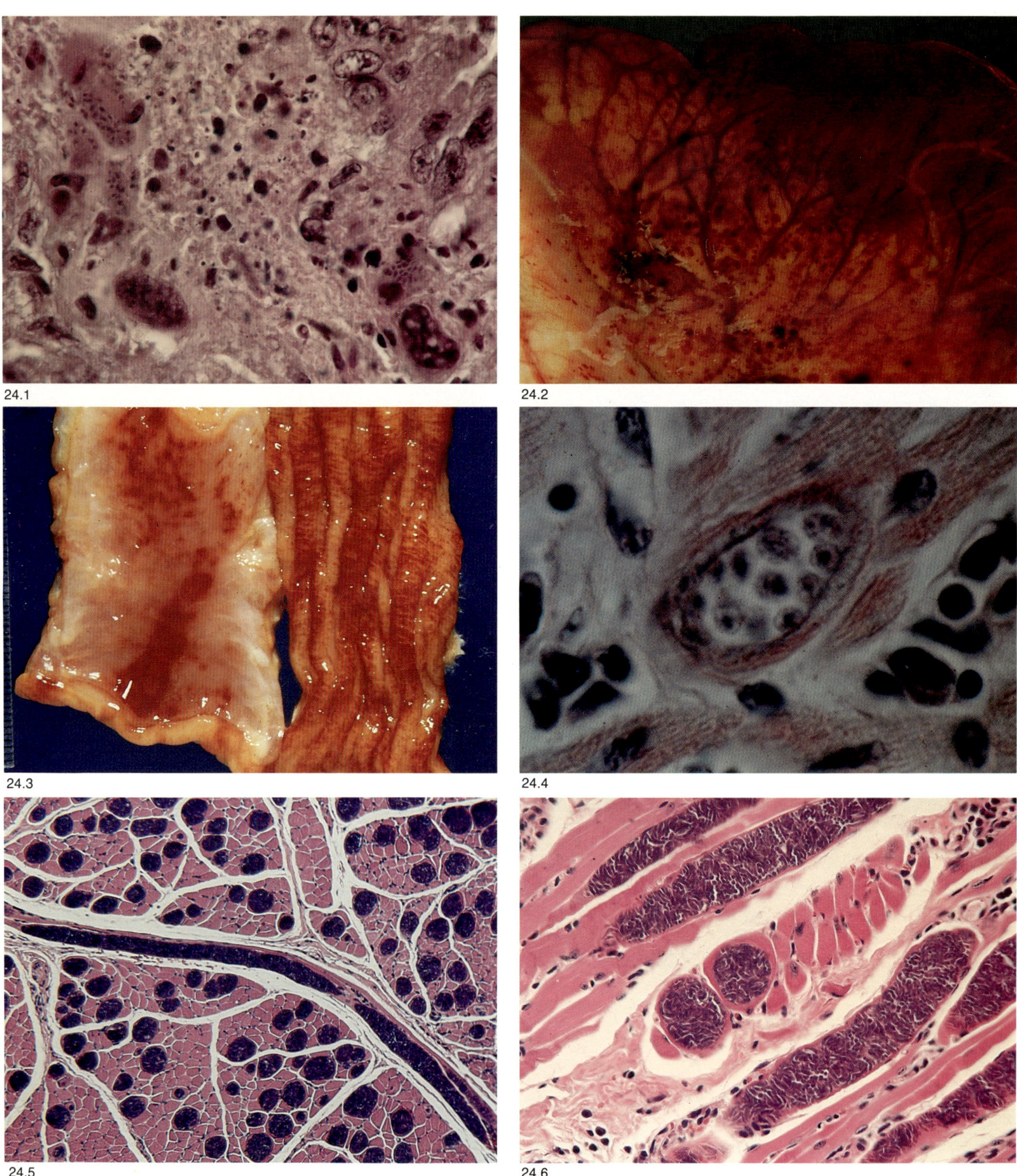

Color plate 24.—*Sarcocystis cruzi* (syn., *S. bovicanis*) of bovines: 24.1, Placental lamina propria of cow with numerous free and intracellular merozoites and immature meronts in area of necrosis, X 630 (84-9522). 24.2, Heart of calf with hemorrhage of myocardium (84-9506). 24.3, Intestine of calf with hemorrhage in serosa (left) and mucosa (right) (84-9524). 24.4, Heart of calf with immature sarcocyst containing globular immature metrocytes, X 630 (84-9525). 24.5, Tongue of calf with numerous basophilic, mature, intramuscular, and microscopic sarcocysts, X 250 (84-9526). 24.6, Higher magnification of mature sarcocysts with longitudinal and cross sections of sarcocysts, X 250 (84-9527).

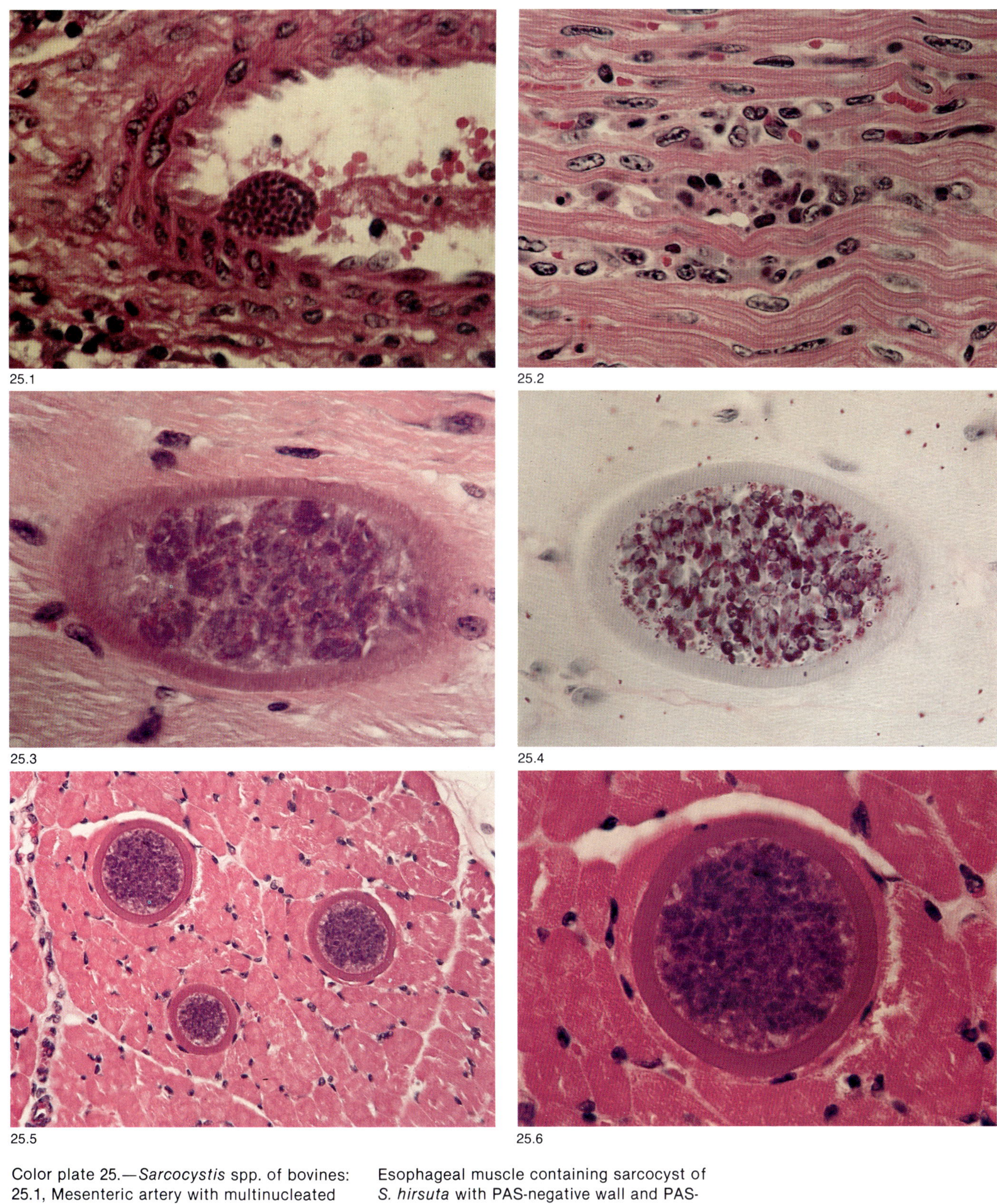

25.1

25.2

25.3

25.4

25.5

25.6

Color plate 25.—*Sarcocystis* spp. of bovines: 25.1, Mesenteric artery with multinucleated first generation meront of *S. hirsuta* (syn., *S. bovifelis*) protruding into lumen, X 630 (84-9509). 25.2, Myocardium with second generation meront of *S. hirsuta* surrounded by inflammatory cells, X 630 (84-9510). 25.3, Esophageal muscle with thick-walled sarcocyst of *S. hirsuta,* X 630 (84-9511). 25.4, Esophageal muscle containing sarcocyst of *S. hirsuta* with PAS-negative wall and PAS-positive granules in zoites, X 630, PASH stain (84-9512). 25.5, Tongue muscle with three thick-walled sarcocysts of *S. hominis* (syn., *S. bovihominis*), X 250 (84-9513). 25.6, Higher magnification of sarcocyst of *S. hominis*, X 630 (84-9514).

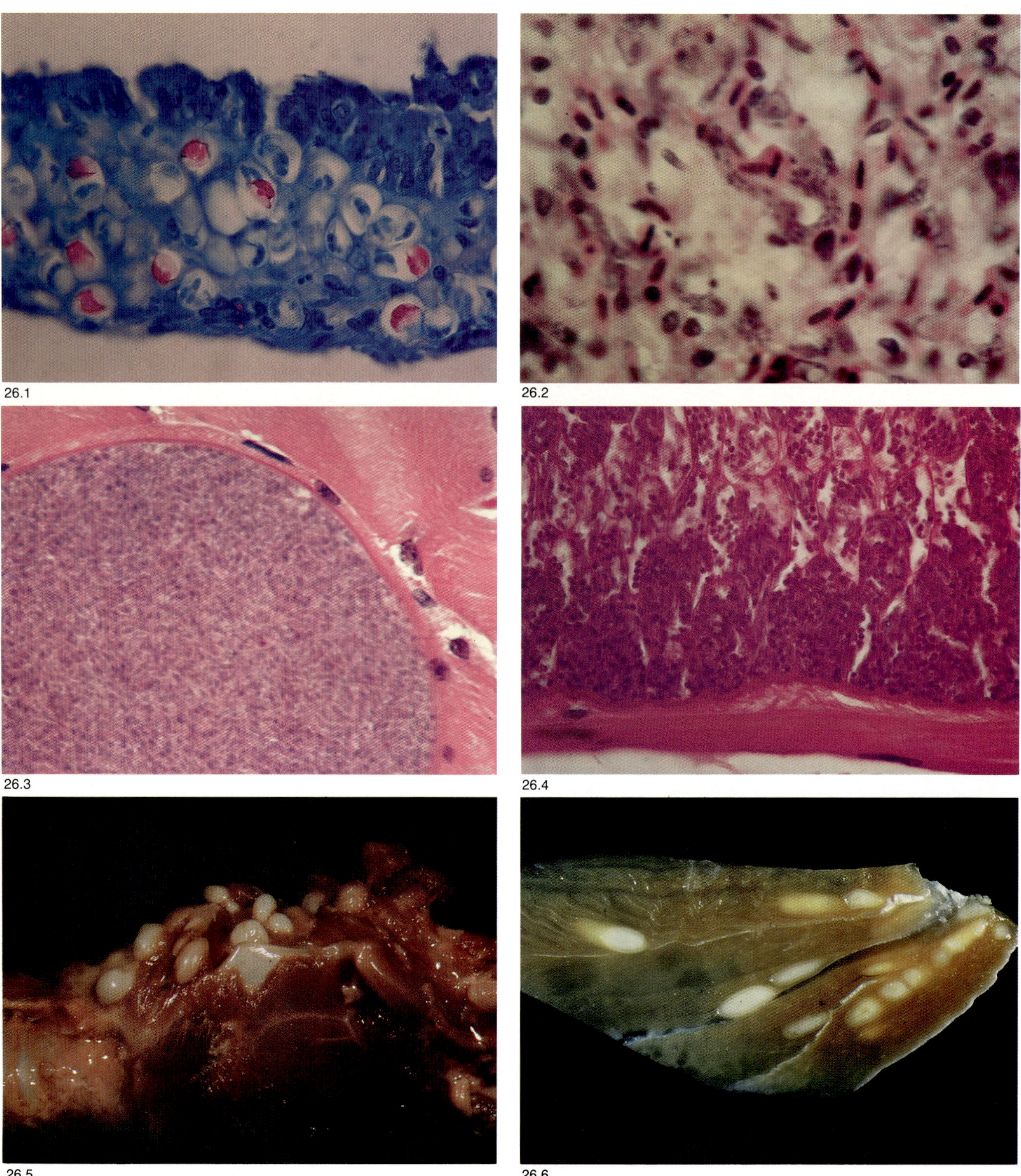

Color plate 26.—*Sarcocystis* spp. of various animals: 26.1, Small intestine of rattlesnake; note acid-fastness of mature sporozoites, X 630, acid-fast stain (84-9528). 26.2, Lung of penguin with sinuous schizont in endothelium of capillary, X 1000 (84-5253). 26.3, Muscle of seal containing mature sarcocyst, X 1000 (84-9578). 26.4, Muscle of cat containing sarcocyst, X 630 (84-9579). 26.5, Trachea of sheep containing large sarcocysts (84-9527). 26.6, Muscle of bird containing large sarcocysts (84-9530).

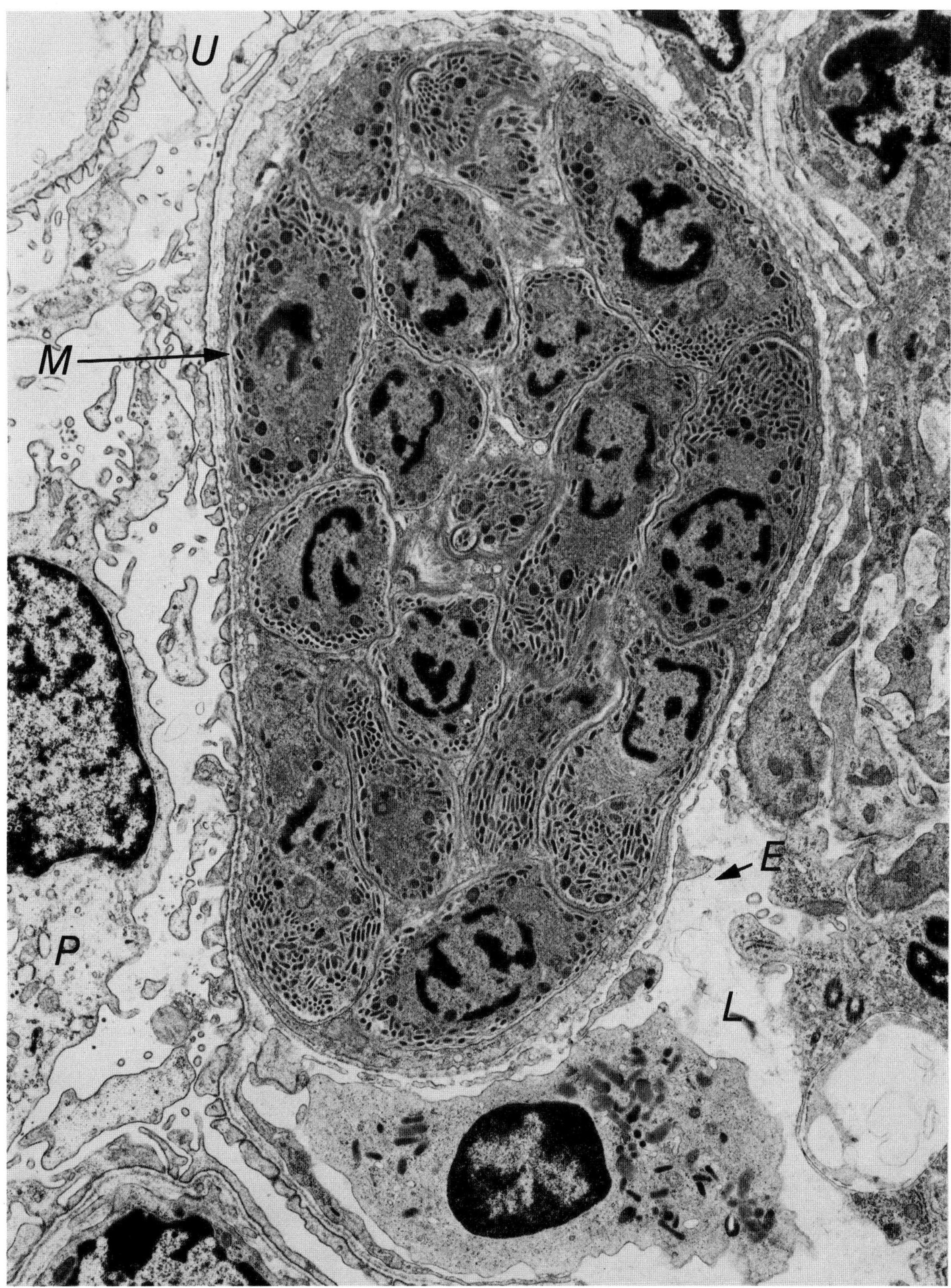

Black and white plate 3.—Electron micrograph of *Sarcocystis* of sheep. Mature second generation schizont of *S. tenella* with several merozoites (*M*) in glomerular capillary and with schizont in direct contact with host cell cytoplasm, without a parasitophorous vacuole, X 12,300. *E*, endothelial cell; *L*, lumen of glomerular capillary; *P*, podocyte; *U*, urinary space. Diagnostically, it is important to recognize that *Sarcocystis* schizonts are distinguished from other coccidia by lack of a parasitophorous vacuole.

Frenkelia

Coccidia of the genus *Frenkelia* have an obligatory two-host life cycle involving a rodent intermediate host (prey) and a raptorial bird definitive host (predator). Except for marked morphologic differences in the cyst stage, the life cycle is nearly identical to that of the *Sarcocystis* spp.

Rodents are infected by ingestion of sporulated oocysts (CP27.1) or sporocysts. Merogony occurs in the rodent liver (CP27.2), and tissue cysts are found in the central nervous system (CP27.3-27.6). Mature tissue cysts can be macroscopic. They are multilobulated and surrounded by a thin wall, with many thousands of slender bradyzoites, which are infectious to the definitive host. After ingestion, bradyzoites enter the intestinal cells and form gametes, which develop into oocysts after fertilization. Oocysts sporulate in situ and are shed in the feces.

Lesions are primarily associated with development of first generation meronts in the liver of rodents. Characteristic lesions include hepatic necrosis and perivascular cellular infiltration in numerous organs. Growth of tissue cysts in the central nervous system may result in pressure necrosis of surrounding neural tissue, with a resultant resorptive inflammatory response.

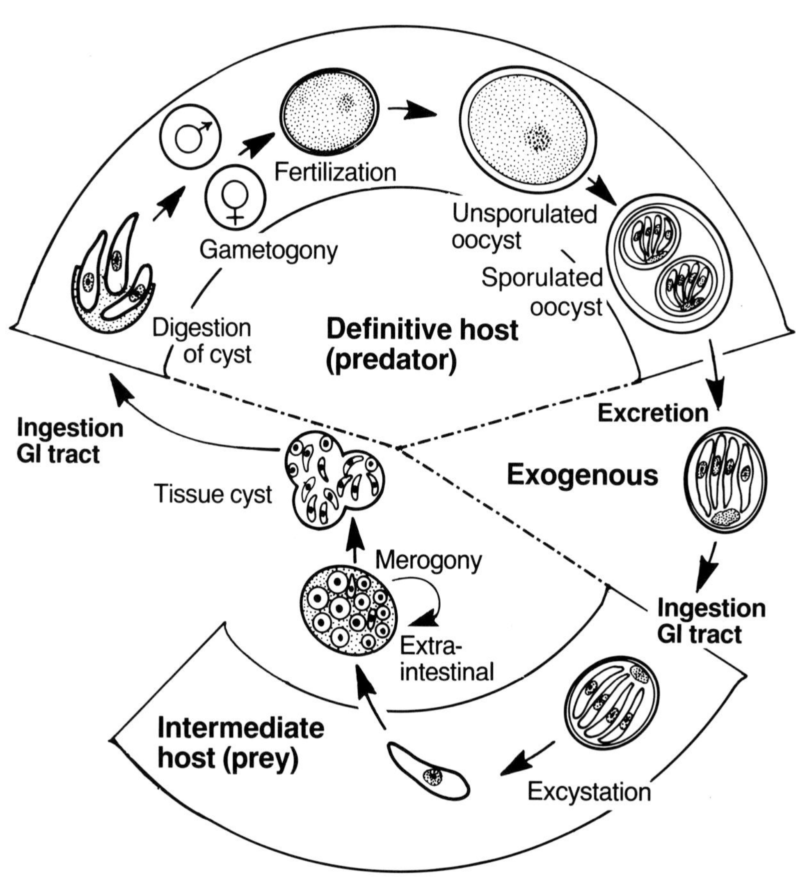

Frenkelia

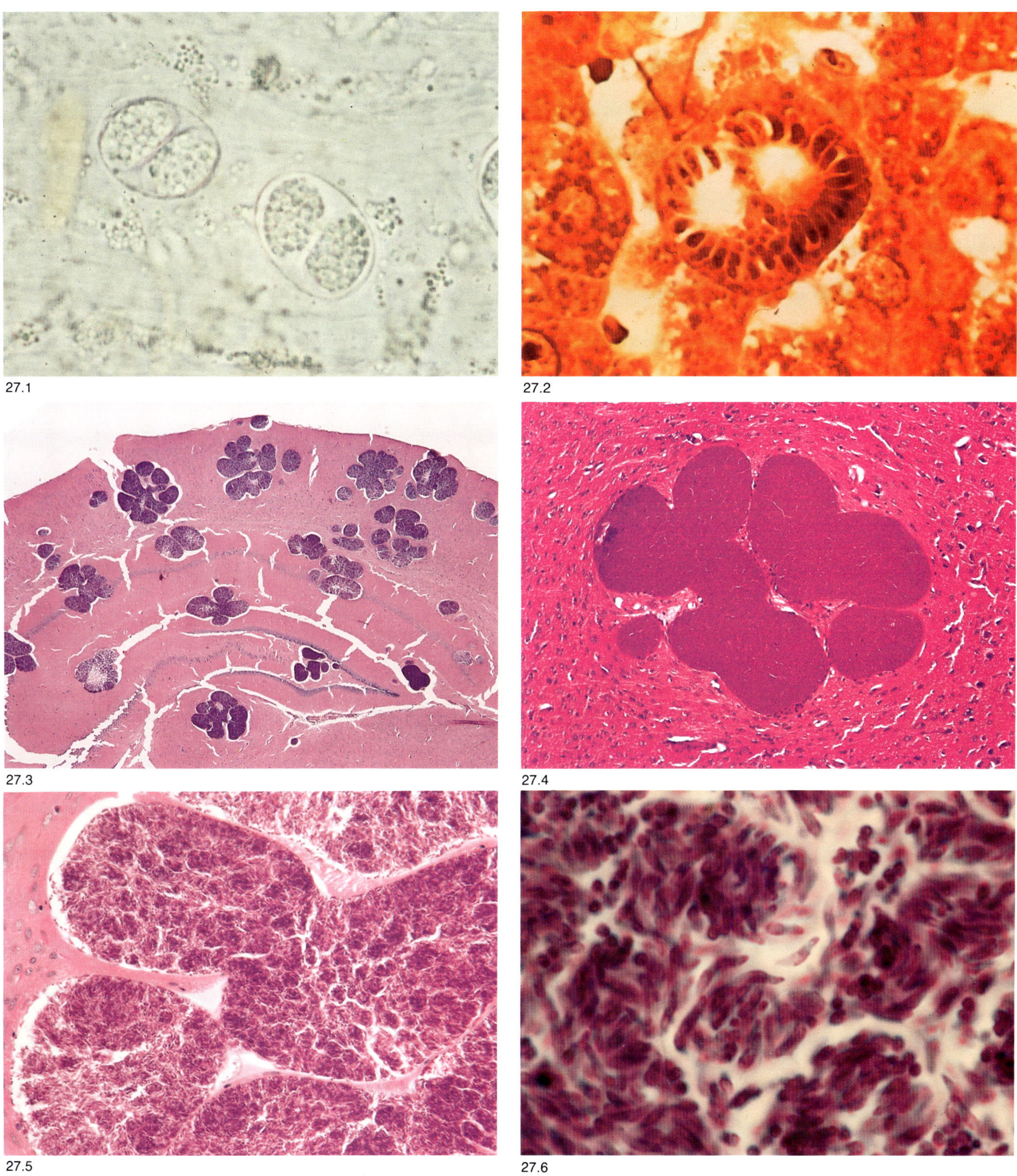

Color plate 27.—*Frenkelia microti* of birds and rodents: 27.1, Feces of European buzzard (*Buteo buteo*) with oocyst stages of *F. microti,* X 630, unstained (84-9438). 27.2, Liver of short-tailed vole (*Microtus agrestis*) containing meront of *F. microti* with peripheral merozoites, X 1000, stain unknown (84-9439). 27.3, Brain of vole (*M. modestus*) naturally infected with numerous lobulated cysts, X 25 (84-9440). 27.4, Higher magnification of 27.3, X 100 (84-9441). 27.5, Higher magnification of cyst, X 250, PASH stain (84-9442). 27.6, Higher magnification of bradyzoites in cyst, X 1500, PASH stain (84-9443).

Besnoitia

Coccidia of the genus *Besnoitia* have been found primarily in bovids in Africa, Asia, and southern Europe, equids in Africa and Mexico, reindeer and caribou in North America, rodents and opossums in the United States, and lizards and opossums in Central America. All these animals are infected with the cyst stage and therefore appear to be intermediate hosts. However, few life cycles are known. Cats have been definitive hosts for three species of *Besnoitia.* Cats shed unsporulated oocysts in the feces. Oocysts sporulate, resembling those of *Isospora* (see chart, p. 20). On ingestion of sporulated oocysts by a susceptible intermediate host, sporozoites excyst and multiply asexually into clusters of fusiform cells (tachyzoites) that initiate cyst development in connective tissue (CP28.3, 28.5, 28.6, 29.1-29.3). These cysts are spherical, white, glistening, and thick walled. They contain many thousands of PAS-positive bradyzoites and grow to several millimeters in diameter (CP28.3, 29.4). The wall is often 10 μm thick or thicker and may contain several host cell nuclei (CP28.6, 29.2, 29.6). Cysts develop in con-nective tissue throughout the body but especially in the skin, conjunctiva, mesentery, and scrotum. On ingestion of cysts by the definitive host, bradyzoites are released and initiate merogony and then gametogony and oocyst formation in the small intestine (CP28.1, 28.2).

Acute lesions of besnoitiosis are associated with multiplication of tachyzoites in experimental infections and chronic lesions with the cyst stage in natural infections. Acute lesions are characterized by necrosis of infected tissue. Chronic lesions result from displacement of normal tissue by cysts (CP29.1, 29.3) and granulomatous inflammation associated with rupture of cysts. Most often there is no inflammatory reaction.

A protozoan parasite, morphologically similar to the cyst stage of *Besnoitia,* infects knots (*Calidris canutus*), migratory birds in the family Scolopacidae, with sometimes fatal effects. Cysts are found in arteries of several organs. Endaortitis, as well as endarteritis of mesenteric and muscular arteries, is the principal lesion (CP30).

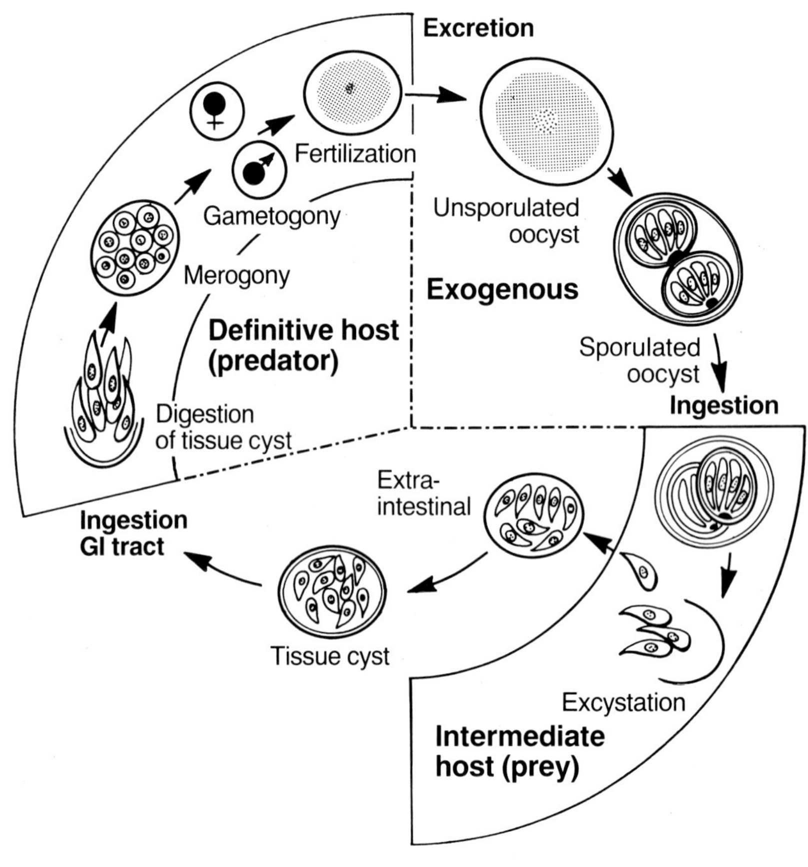

Besnoitia

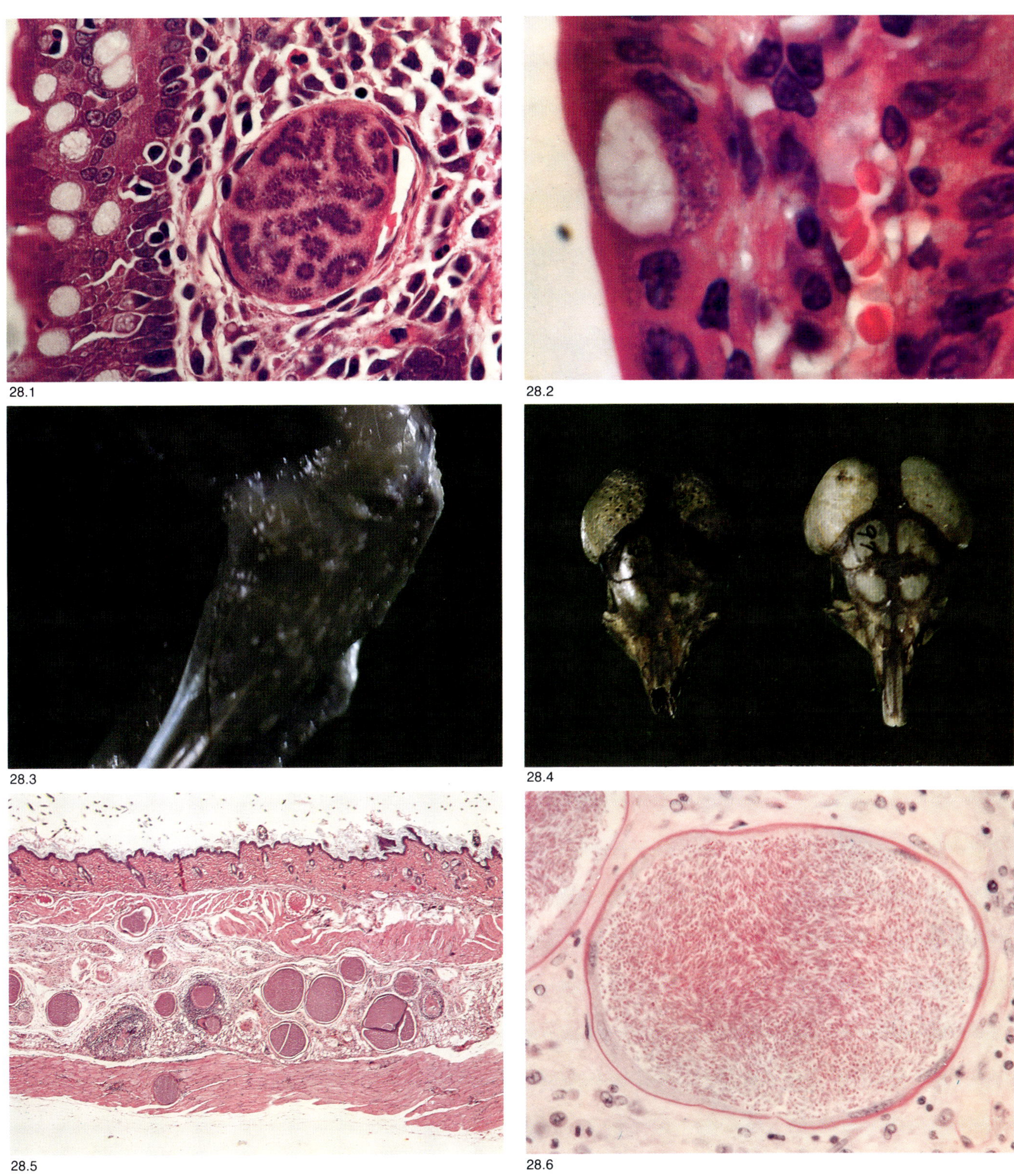

Color plate 28.—*Besnoitia* spp. of animals:
28.1, Small intestine of cat with schizont of
B. wallacei, X 630 (84-9444). 28.2, Small intestine of cat with gamont of *B. wallacei* in
goblet cell, X 1500 (84-9445). 28.3, Hindleg of
kangaroo rat (*Dipodomys ordii*) with
numerous white, raised, subcutaneous cysts
of *B. jellisoni* (84-9446). 28.4, Skulls of
kangaroo rats showing uninfected skull
(right) and infected skull (left) with perforations in mastoid bones due to cysts of *B.
jellisoni* (84-9447). 28.5, Skin of mouse with
cysts of *B. jellisoni* in subcutaneous tissue, X
25 (84-9448). 28.6, Higher magnification of
cyst of *B. jellisoni* with host cell nuclei in
cyst wall, X 400, PASH stain (84-9449).

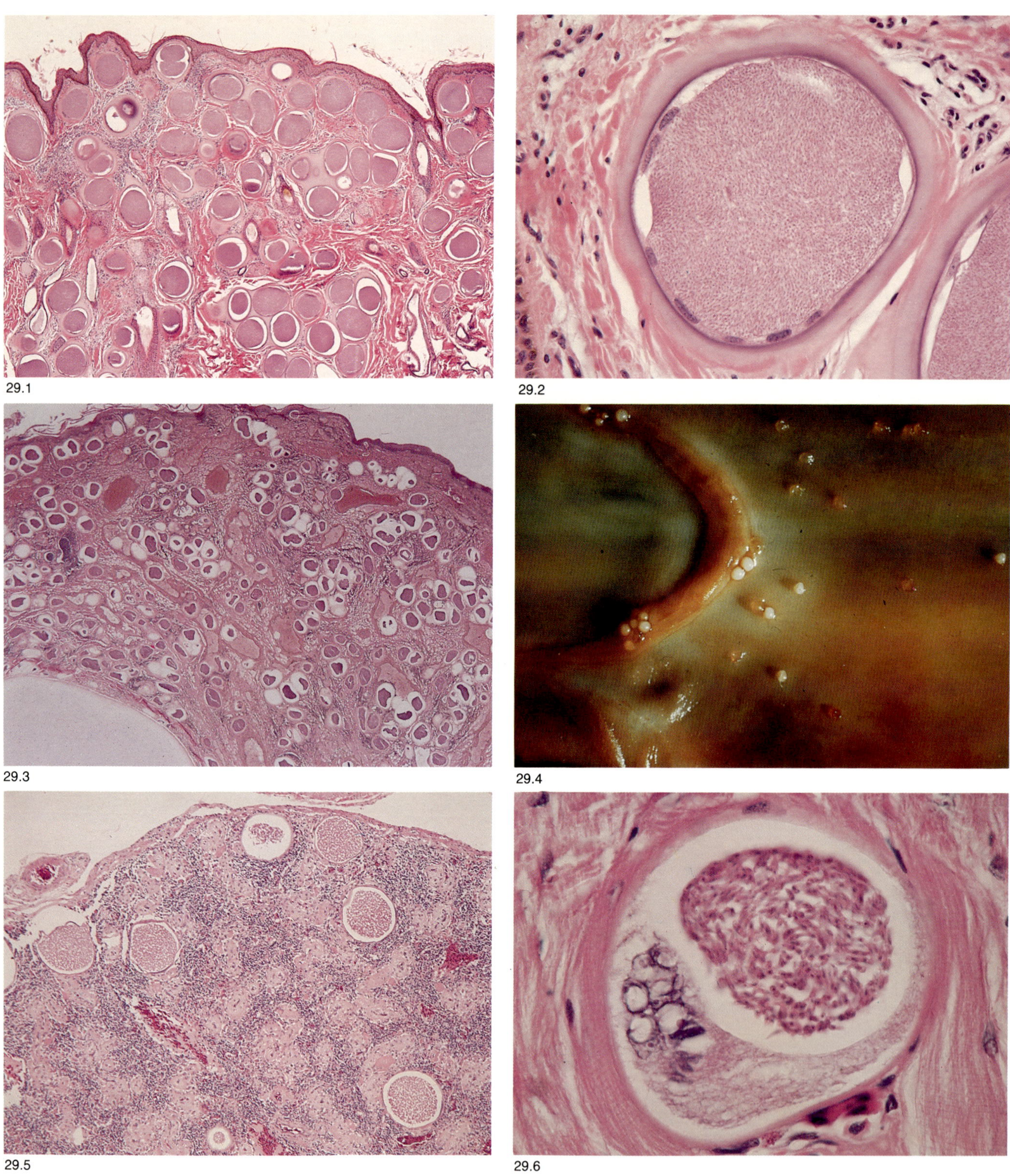

Color plate 29.—*Besnoitia* spp. of animals: 29.1, Skin of ox with numerous cysts of *B. besnoiti* in dermis, X 25 (84-9450). 29.2, Higher magnification of cyst of *B. besnoiti* with hypertrophy and increased number of host cell nuclei in wall of cyst, X 250 (84-9451). 29.3, Eyelid of caribou with numerous cysts of *B. tarandi* in dermis, X 15 (84-5288). 29.4, Jugular vein of blue wildebeest with numerous *Besnoitia* sp. cysts protruding into lumen (84-9452). 29.5, Spleen of spotted lizard with numerous cysts of *Besnoitia* sp., X 60 (84-9453). 29.6, Myocardium of spotted lizard with host cell nuclei in cyst wall (lower left) and numerous bradyzoites (upper right), X 630 (84-9454).

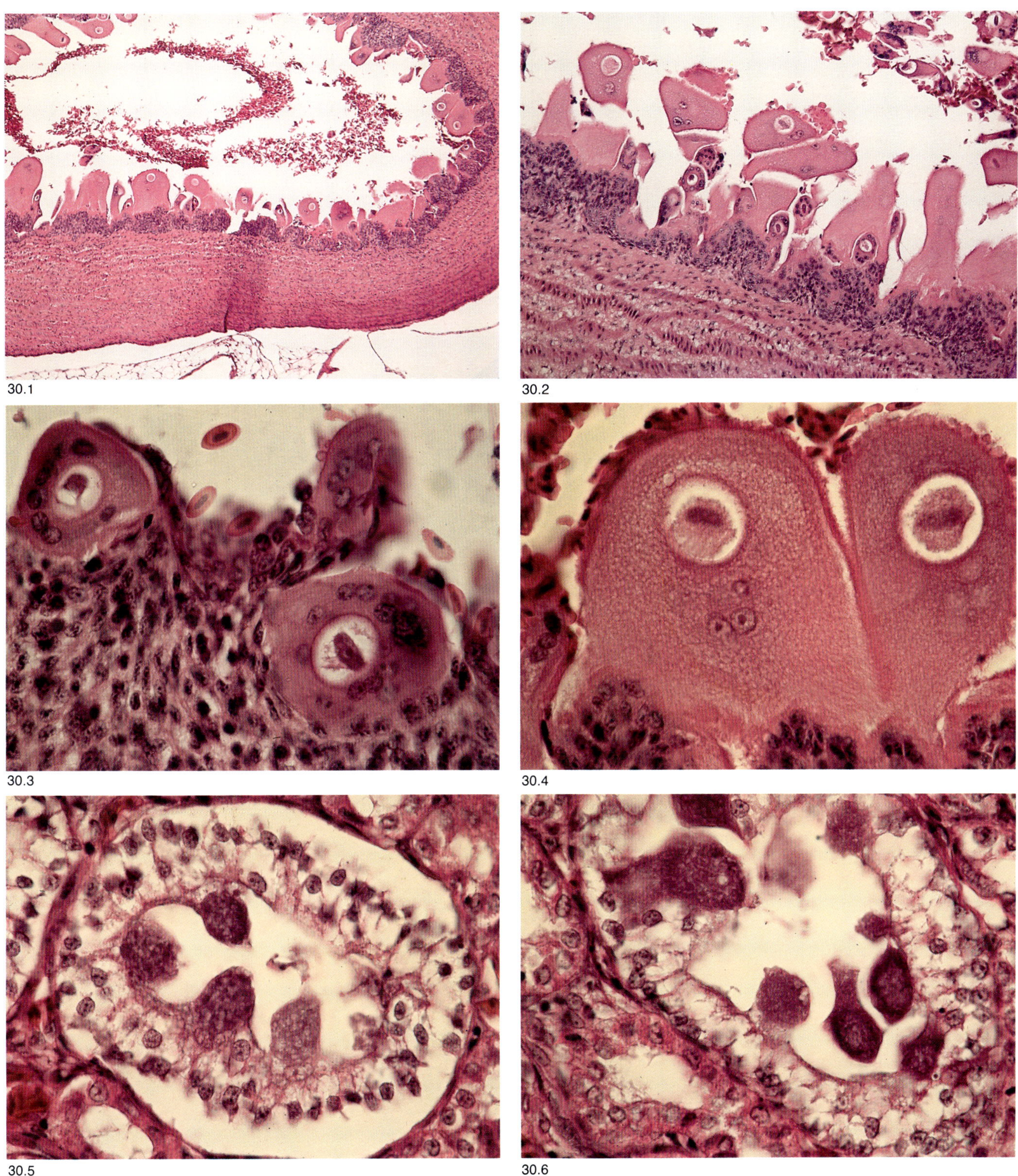

30.1

30.2

30.3

30.4

30.5

30.6

Color plate 30.—*Besnoitia*-like organism of knots: 30.1, Mesenteric artery with organisms in hypertrophied endothelial cells protruding into lumen, X 60 (84-9455). 30.2, Higher magnification of same artery, X 160 (84-9456). 30.3, High magnification showing numerous host cell nuclei surrounding vacuole containing uninucleate organism, X 630 (84-9457). 30.4, High magnification showing elongate basophilic nucleus of parasite within vacuole in host cells, X 630 (84-9458). 30.5, Kidney tubules with multinucleated meronts in cuboidal cells protruding into lumen, X 630 (84-9459). 30.6, Kidney tubule with numerous meronts, X 630 (84-9460).

Toxoplasma and *Hammondia*

The coccidium *Toxoplasma gondii* infects all warm-blooded animals, including humans. Felids (both domestic and wild) are the only definitive hosts; felids and nonfelids are intermediate hosts. *Toxoplasma* can be transmitted to intermediate hosts via oocysts in feline feces, via cysts in host tissues (meat), and via tachyzoites transplacentally. Unsporulated oocysts ($\sim$10 μm in diameter) in feline feces (CP31.2) sporulate outside the body and become infectious. On ingestion, sporozoites excyst and multiply in the intestine and associated lymph nodes as tachyzoites. Tachyzoites (rapidly multiplying, crescent-shaped zoites, 4 to 6 μm long) multiply by endodyogeny (two progeny forming within a parent cell) for numerous generations, spreading through tissues and circulation, and then encyst. Cysts persist most frequently in the brain, liver, muscles, and retina. They are usually spherical or elongate (10 to 100 μm long), thin-walled structures containing a few to several hundred slender PAS-positive bradyzoites or slowly multiplying zoites (CP32.3-32.5). Cysts ingested by a nonfeline host release bradyzoites, which become tachyzoites, and the cycle is repeated. Infection by either oocysts or cysts during pregnancy can result in transplacental infection of the fetus with tachyzoites.

Toxoplasma is transmitted to cats that ingest either sporulated oocysts or tissues infected with tachyzoites, but the most common source of infection is ingestion of tissues containing cysts. On ingestion of cysts, bradyzoites released in the gastrointestinal tract initiate an enteroepithelial cycle of asexual and sexual multiplication (CP31.1), followed by oocyst development and shedding of unsporulated oocysts with feces. An extraintestinal cycle, like that seen in nonfelids, also occurs in cats.

Tachyzoite multiplication results in focal necrosis (CP32.1, 32.2), the most characteristic lesion of toxoplasmosis. Inflammation usually follows necrosis. Pneumonitis is the predominant lesion in fatal toxoplasmosis in cats and dogs (CP31.4); placental necrosis with white flecks or multiple white, chalky, necrotic nodules (CP32.1) and associated abortion predominate in sheep (CP33) and goats. Histologically, this necrosis is confined to the cotyledons where individual and small groups of tachyzoites are often difficult to recognize among degenerating host cells. Encephalomyelitis is the predominant lesion in sheep and goat fetuses.

Diagnosis of *Toxoplasma* is also aided by serologic tests and by bioassay or xenodiagnosis in mice.

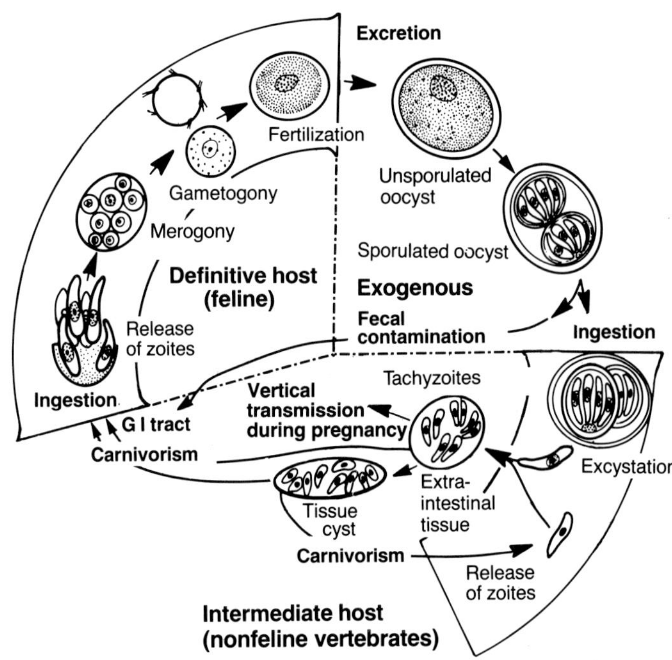

Toxoplasma

Hammondia hammondi is a nonpathogenic coccidian of cats closely related to *T. gondii*. Its life cycle and structure are essentially the same as those of *T. gondii* with the following exceptions: (1) *H. hammondi* has no extraintestinal cycle in the cat; (2) intermediate hosts become infected only by ingestion of oocysts; and (3) definitive hosts become infected only by ingestion of cysts in tissues of intermediate hosts (CP32.6). Differentiation of *H. hammondi* from *T. gondii* must be based on a life-cycle study.

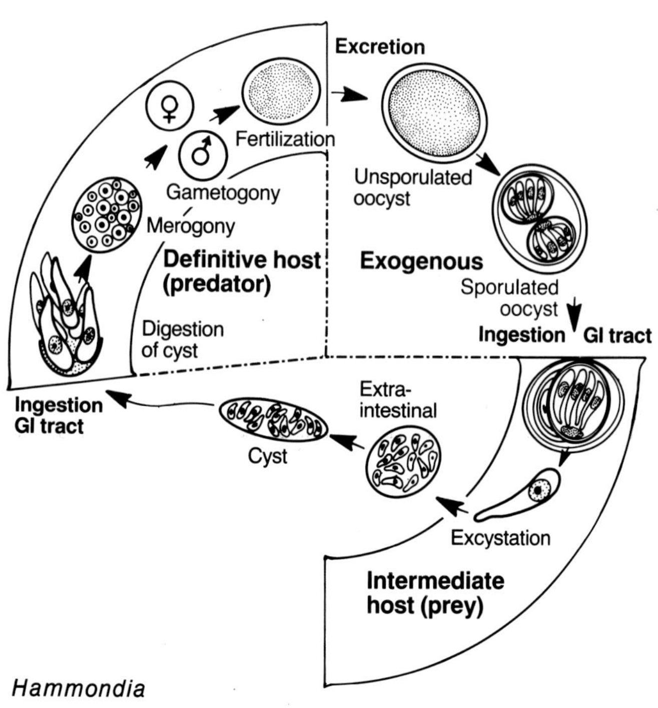

Hammondia

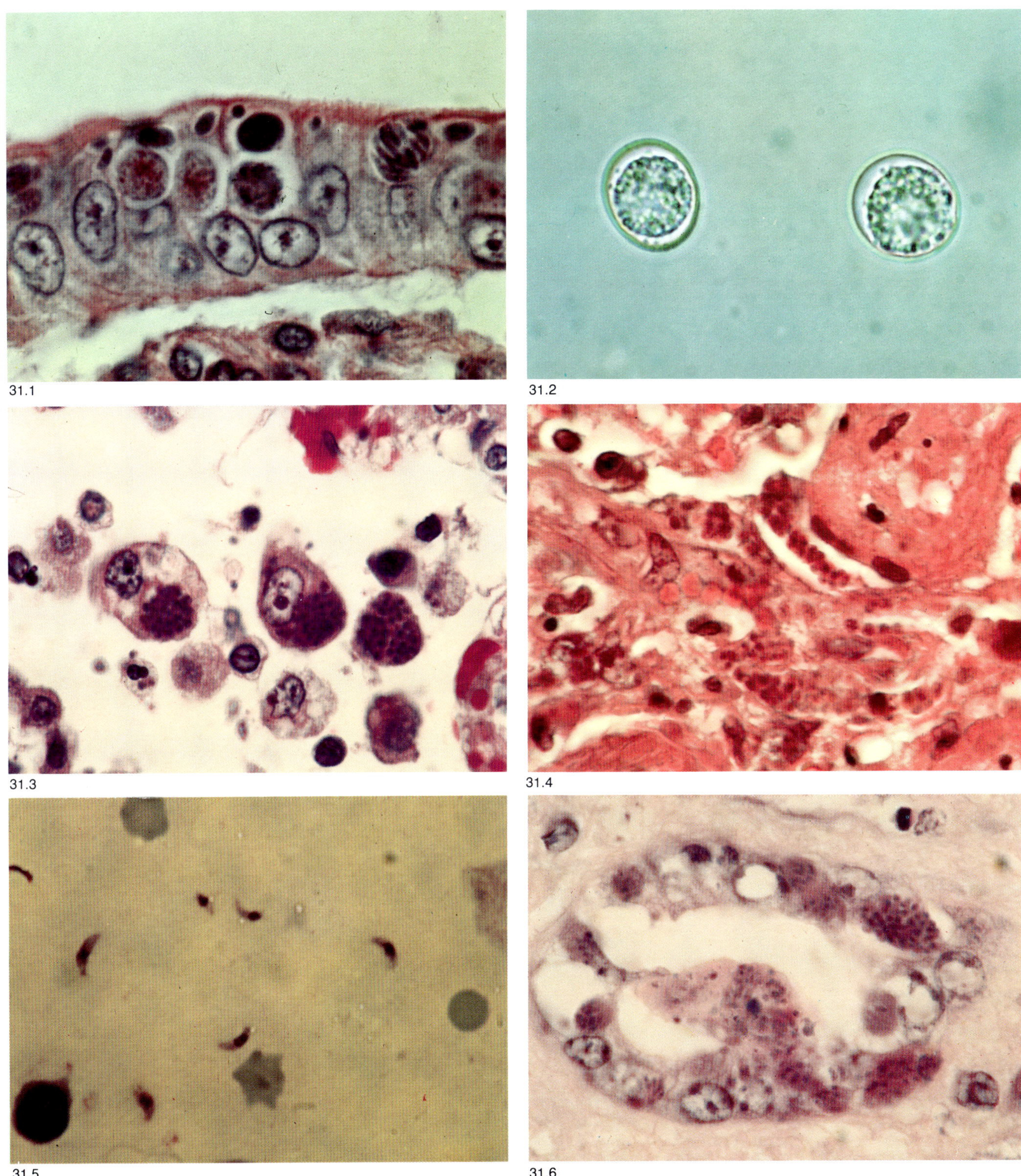

Color plate 31.—*Toxoplasma gondii* of animals: 31.1, Small intestine of cat showing numerous asexual and sexual stages in epithelial cells with macrogametes in two cells (left), microgamont in cell (center), and meront in cell (right), X 1000 (84-9533). 31.2, Feces of cat with two unsporulated oocysts in fecal float, X 1000 (84-9534). 31.3, Lung of cat with numerous tachyzoites in macrophages in alveolar lumen, X 1000 (84-9535). 31.4, Lung of cat containing numerous oval-to-round tachyzoites, each with basophilic nucleus, X 1000 (84-9536). 31.5, Lung of cat with lunate tachyzoites in impression smear, X 1000, Giemsa stain (84-9537). 31.6, Kidney of goat with numerous tachyzoites in tubular epithelium, X 1000 (84-9538).

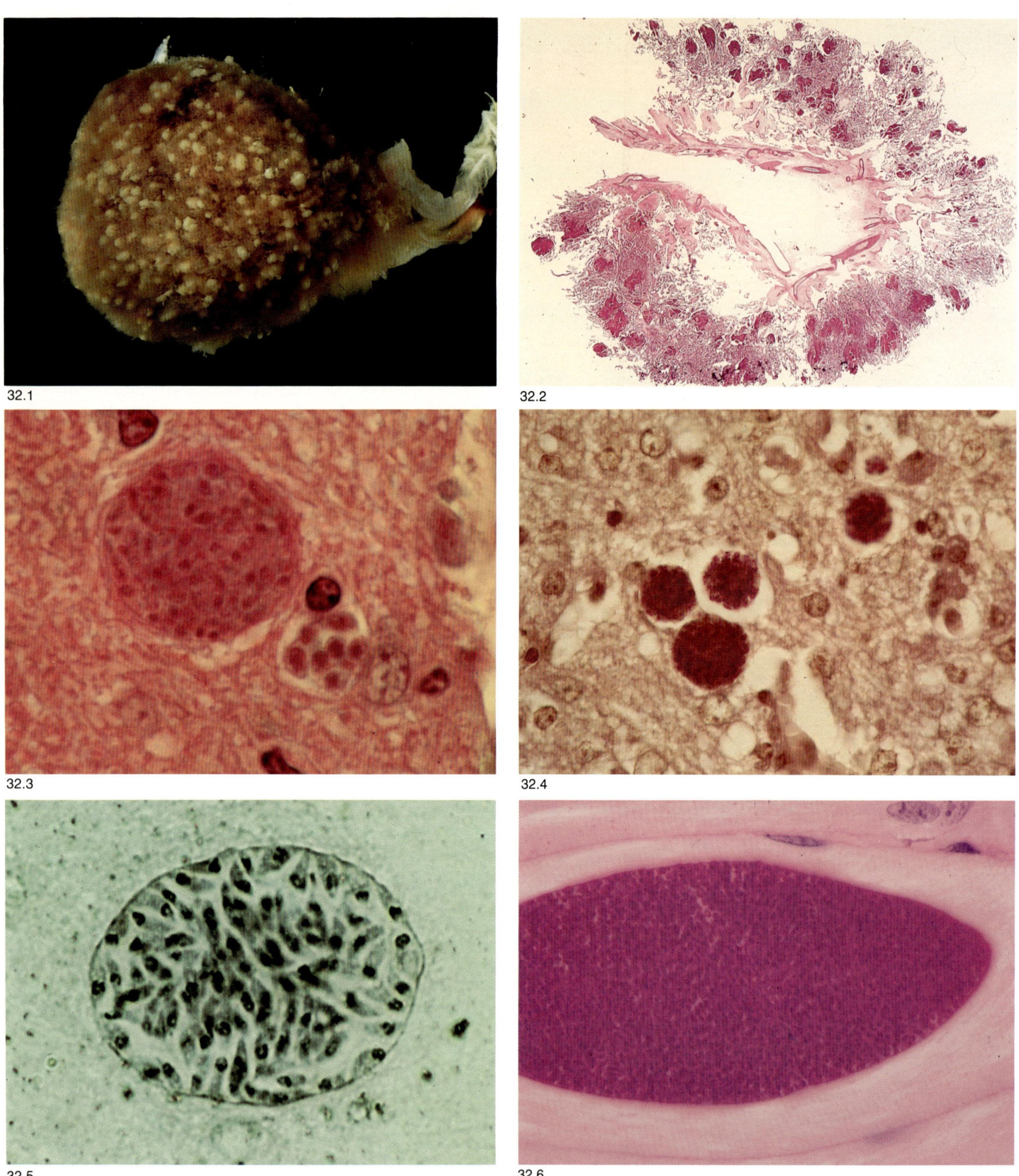

Color plate 32.—*Toxoplasma* and *Hammondia* of animals: 32.1, Placenta of sheep showing cotyledon with numerous yellowish-white necrotic foci in villi (84-9539). 32.2, Placenta of sheep with multifocal necrosis in villi, X 3, PAS stain (84-9540). 32.3, Brain of mouse with cyst (upper left) and group of tachyzoites (lower right), which are larger than bradyzoites, X 1500 (84-9542). 32.4, Brain of mouse containing four cysts with PAS-positive bradyzoites, X 630, PASH stain (84-9543). 32.5, Brain of mouse containing cyst with thin argentophilic wall and numerous bradyzoites with terminal or subterminal nucleus in impression smear, X 1000, Gomori methanamine silver-Giemsa stain (84-9544). 32.6, Skeletal muscle of mouse with *H. hammondi* cyst, X 630, PASH stain (84-9580).

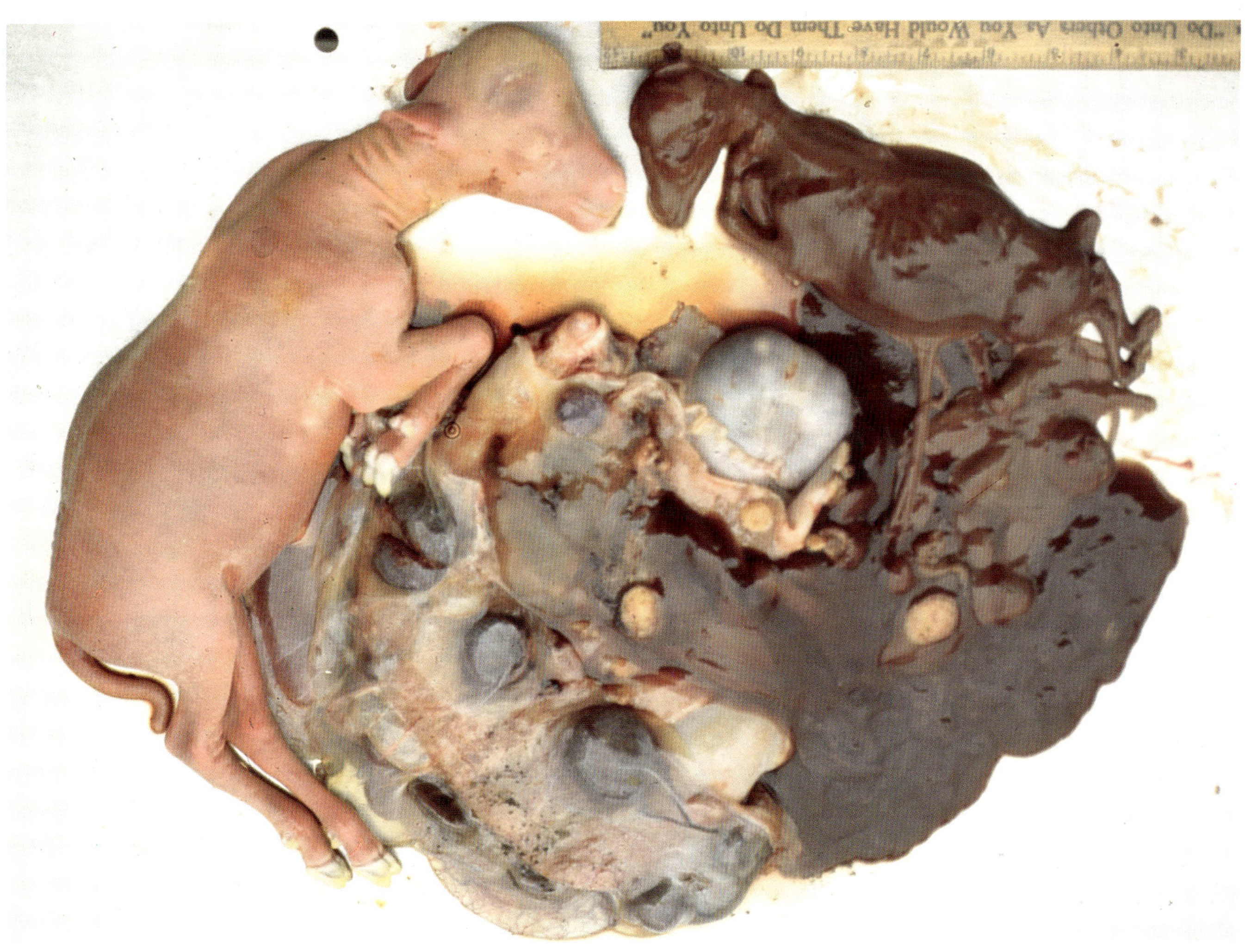

Color plate 33.—*Toxoplasma* abortion of sheep.   Darker lamb and associated fetal membranes are severely autolyzed.   Lighter lamb and associated fetal membranes are not autolyzed.   Lesions, characteristic of *Toxoplasma*, are found in cotyledons of both lambs.   (Scale = 2.5 cm)

Coccidia of Undetermined Taxonomic Status

Coccidia-like organisms have been observed with light and electron microscopy in tissues of horses, cattle, and sheep. The organisms appear morphologically similar to meronts of *Sarcocystis*, but because other stages of the life cycle have not been observed, their taxonomic status remains undetermined. The sources of such infections are not known.

In horses, organisms in the blood vessels and neural cells of the central nervous system have been associated with encephalomyelitis (CP34.1, 34.2). In sheep (CP34.3-34.6) and calves (CP35.1-35.4), a similar organism has been associated with similar lesions.

In aborted fetal horses, organisms in undetermined cells in the lung (CP35.5-35.6) appear similar to meronts of *Sarcocystis.*

In dogs, dermal nodules contain coccidian stages within macrophages (CP36.4, 36.5). They are located in the dermis and appear similar to *Caryospora.*

In birds, tiny merozoitelike stages have been found in the intestine. Some appear to be intracellular and others extracellular (CP36.6).

Coccidia of the genus *Calyptospora* have been reported only in fish (CP36.1), where the oocysts sporulate in situ in the liver. Oocysts resembling those of *Calyptospora* have been found in the livers of crocodiles (CP36.2). As in some other genera of coccidia, the sporozoites are acid-fast (CP36.3).

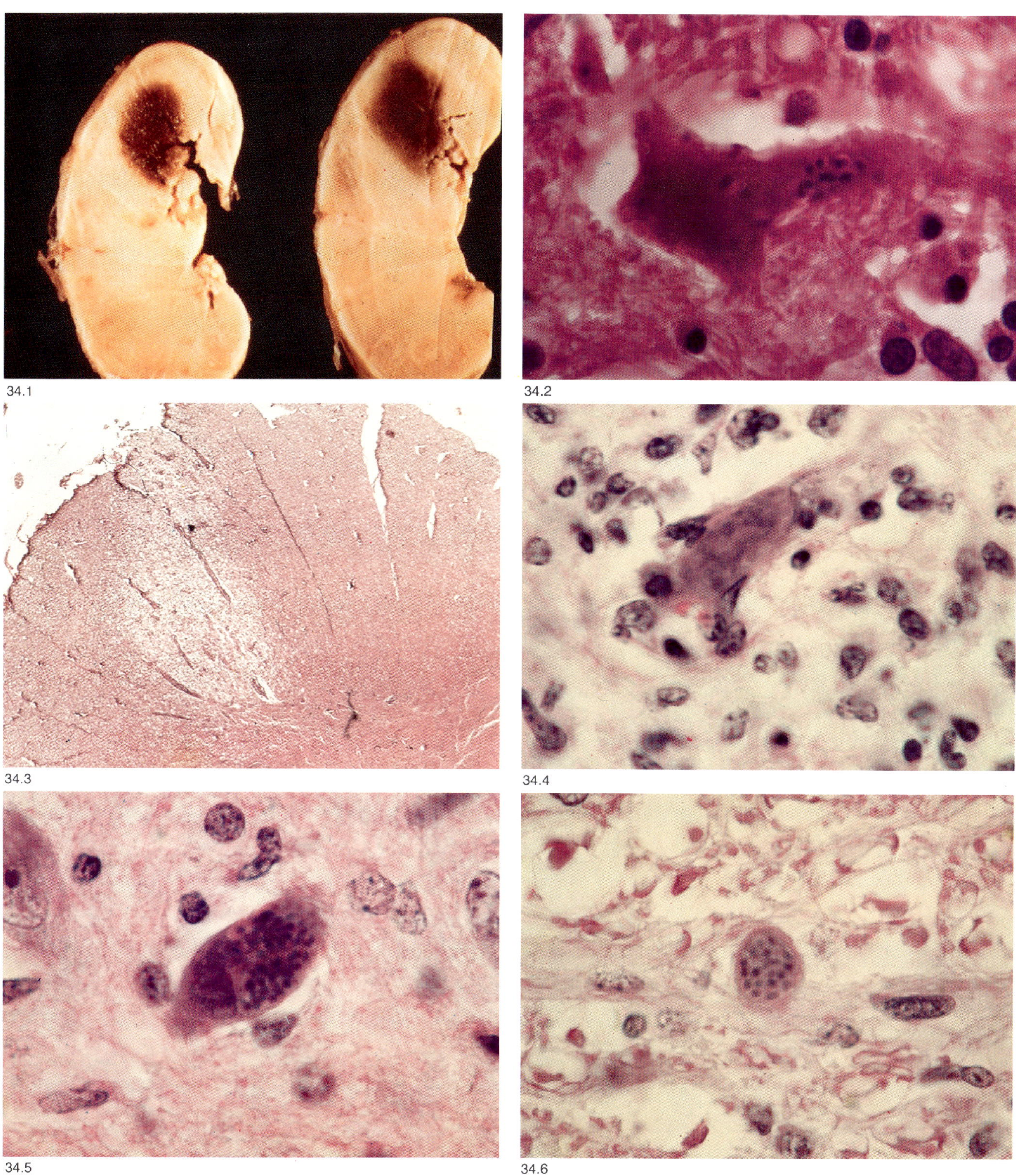

Color plate 34.—Coccidia of undetermined taxonomic status causing encephalomyelitis of domestic animals: 34.1, Medulla oblongata of horse with large dark focal lesion characterized by necrosis (84-9545). 34.2, Spinal cord of horse containing organisms within neuron, X 1000 (84-9546). 34.3, Spinal cord of sheep showing focal necrosis with perivascular infiltration, X 5 (84-9547). 34.4, Cerebrum of 3-week-old lamb with immature meront in capillary, X 1000 (84-9548). 34.5, Cerebrum of lamb in 34.4 containing two meronts within one capillary, immature (left) and mature (right), X 1000 (84-9549). 34.6, Cerebrum of lamb in 34.4 with small multinucleated meront, X 1000 (84-9550).

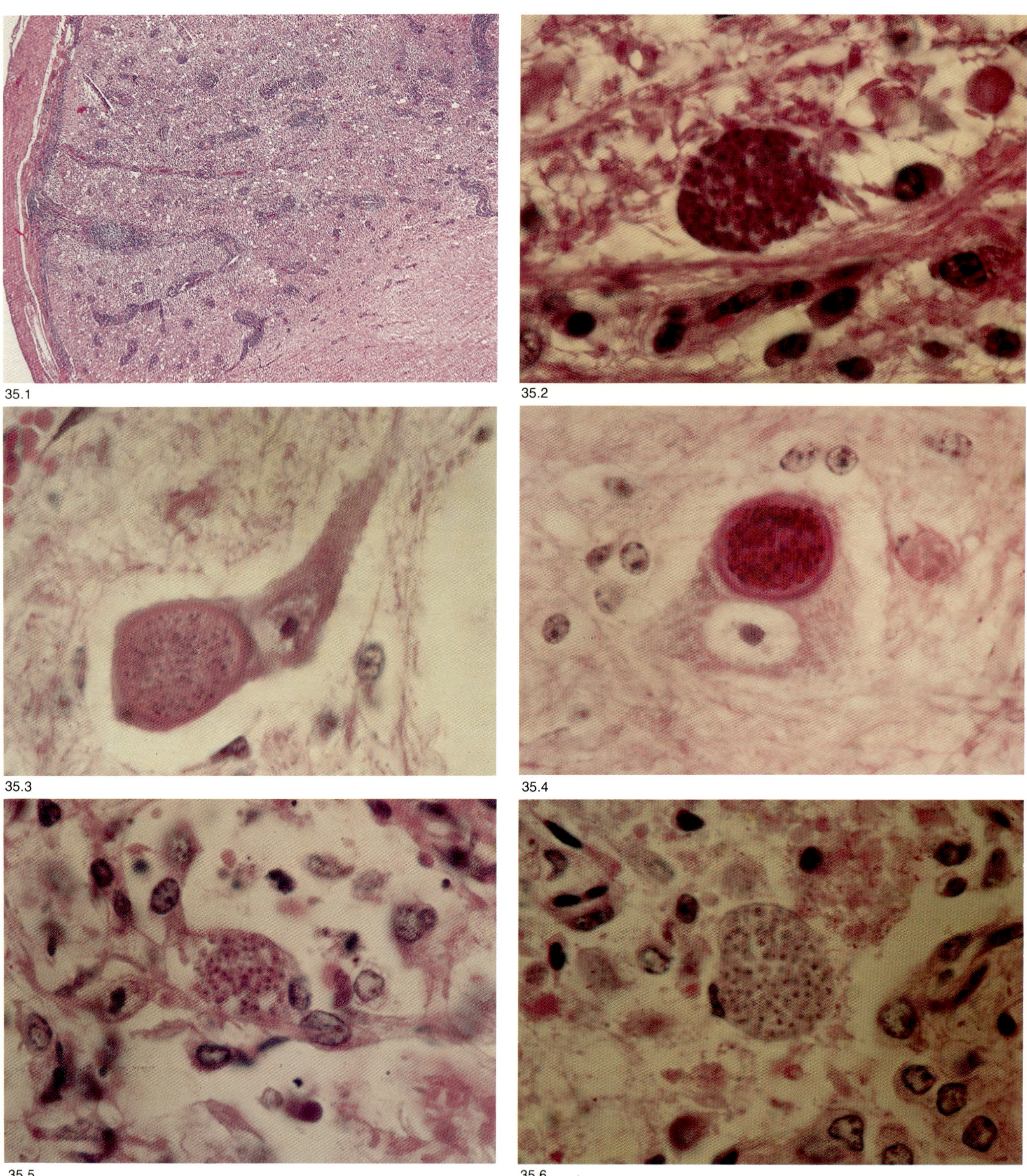

35.1

35.2

35.3

35.4

35.5

35.6

Color plate 35.—Coccidia of undetermined taxonomic status of animals: 35.1, Spinal cord of bovine calf with severe submeningeal perivascular infiltration in white matter, X 25 (84-9551). 35.2, Higher magnification of 35.1 with group of zoites in parenchyma, X 1000 (84-9552). 35.3, Spinal cord of bovine calf containing cystlike structure with numerous zoites within neuron in gray matter, X 1000 (84-9553). 35.4, Spinal cord of calf in 35.3 containing cyst with numerous PAS-positive granules, X 1000, PASH stain (84-9554). 35.5, Fetal lung of horse with numerous organisms in cell protruding into alveolus, X 1000 (84-9555). 35.6, Fetal lung in 35.5 containing cyst with numerous uninucleate PAS-negative zoites, X 1000, PASH stain (84-9556).

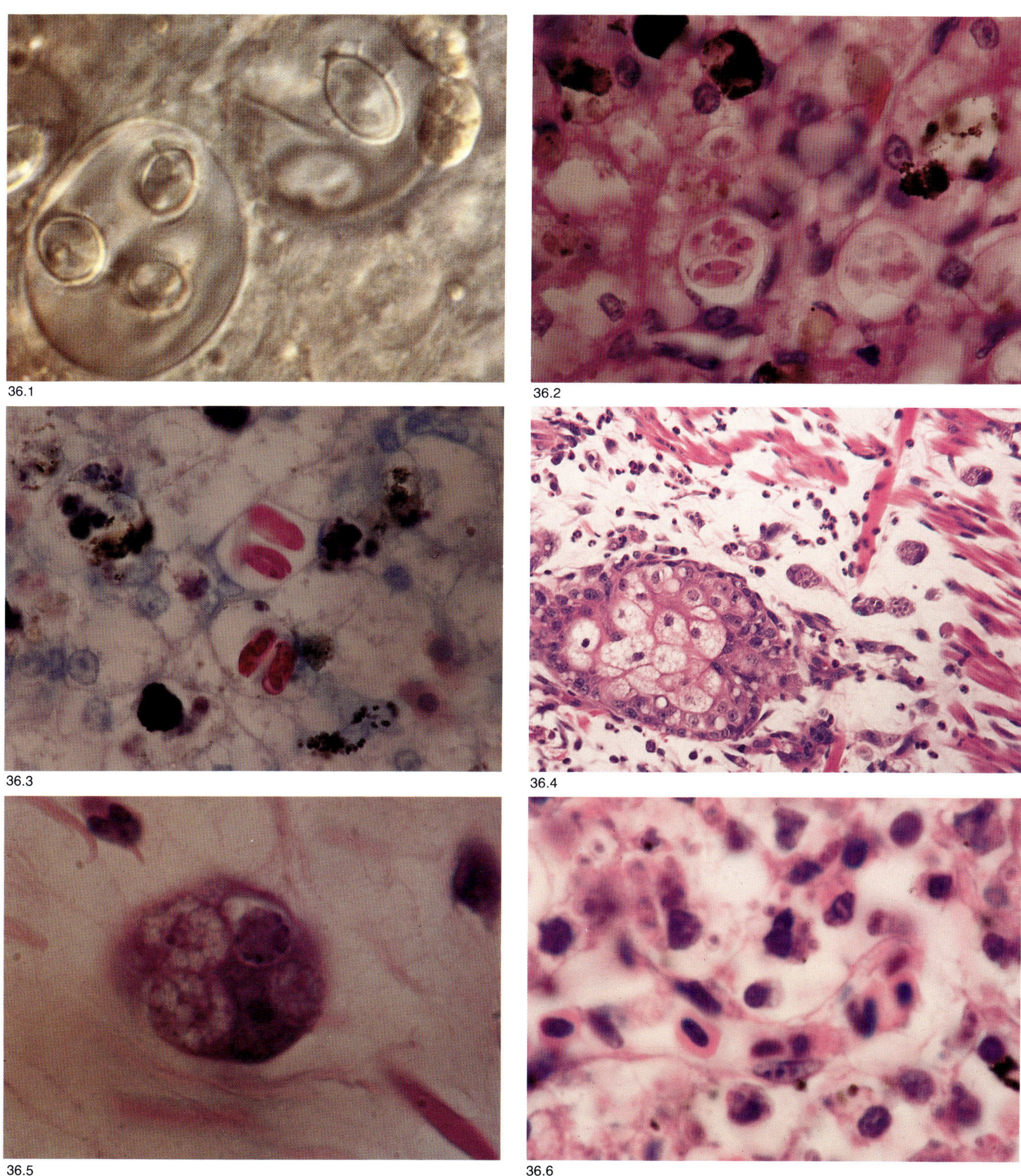

36.1

36.2

36.3

36.4

36.5

36.6

Color plate 36.—*Calyptospora* and organisms of undetermined taxonomic status of animals: 36.1, Liver impression smear of fish; note sporulated oocysts of *C. funduli*, X 2500 (84-9572). 36.2, Liver of crocodile with sporulated oocysts of coccidian perhaps related to *Calyptospora* spp., X 1000 (84-9573). 36.3, Liver of crocodile with coccidia in 36.2 containing acid-fast sporozoites when mature, X 1000, acid-fast stain (84-9574). 36.4, Skin of dog; note gamonts and gametes of coccidian in host cells perhaps related to *Caryospora* spp. (CP20), X 250 (84-9575). 36.5, Skin of dog with host cell nucleus (dark, lower right), three macrogametes, and one microgamont (upper right with peripheral dark nuclei) that may be related to *Caryospora* sp. (see CP20), X 1500 (84-9576). 36.6, Small intestine of finch with tiny organisms intracellularly and extracellularly that may be *Isospora* spp., X 1500 (84-9577).

Klossiella

Klossiella spp. have been identified most commonly in equids, mice, and guinea pigs and to a less extent in bats, opossums, various rodents, and a boa constrictor. Stages of the organism are found in the kidney (CP37). The life cycle is not clearly understood. In epithelial cells of tubules, trophozoites form schizonts and merozoites, and from these schizonts, gametes are thought to form. Fertilized gametes are believed to develop into sporonts, which bud to form sporoblasts (CP37.2, 37.5). Each of these sporoblasts undergoes successive divisions to form sporocysts that contain sporozoites (CP37.3, 37.6). Mature sporocysts are surrounded by a thick wall and pass from the body in the urine. They are thought to be later ingested by another host, and sporozoites, released from the sporocyst, move to the kidney, where they enter epithelial cells and initiate the cycle.

Only heavily parasitized kidneys have gross lesions, which appear as tiny gray foci on the cortical surface. Microscopically these foci are areas of necrosis, with perivascular infiltration of inflammatory cells, especially lymphocytes and histiocytes, and with an increase in interstitial fibroblasts.

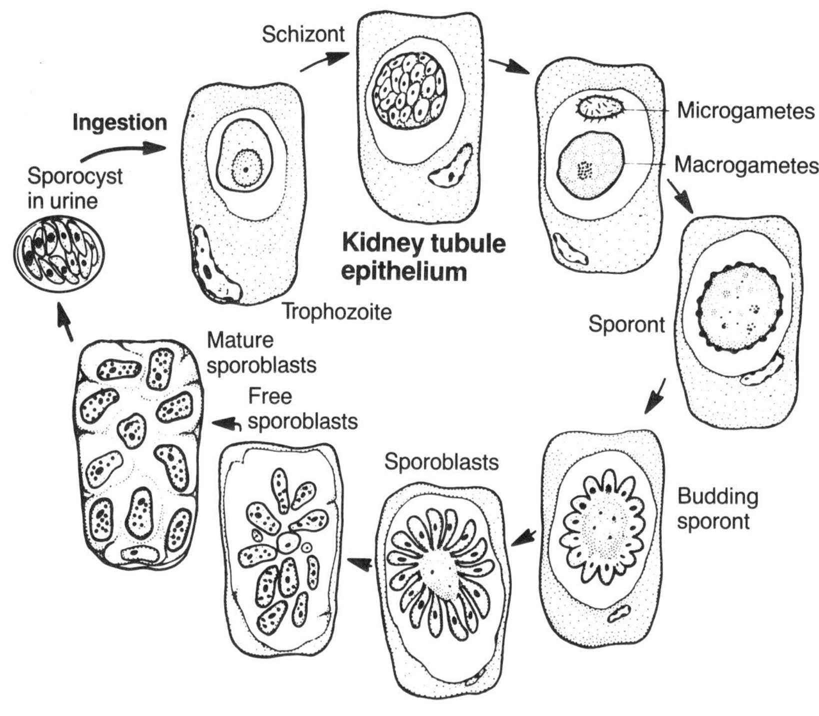

Klossiella

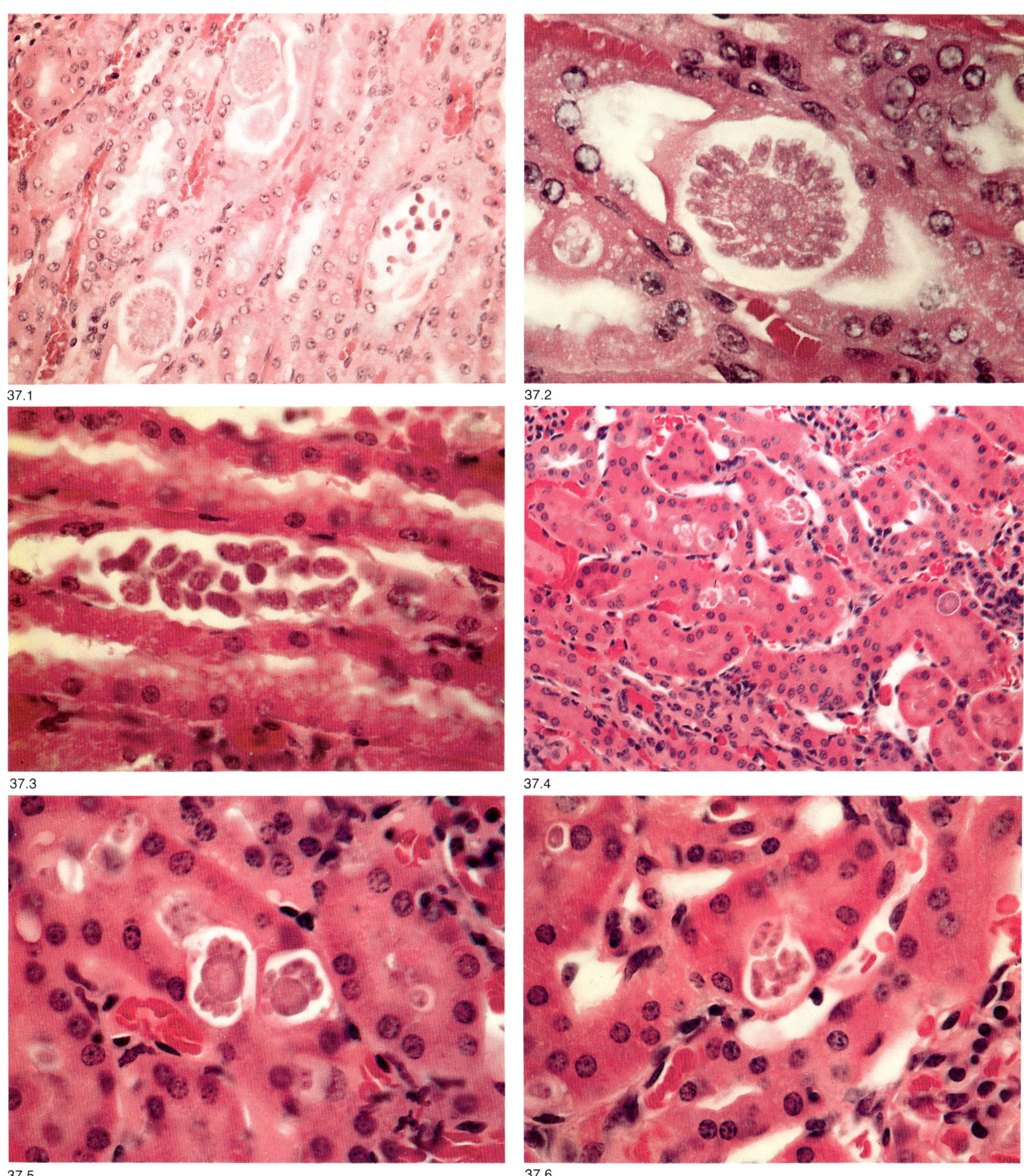

37.1 37.2

37.3 37.4

37.5 37.6

Color plate 37.—*Klossiella* spp. of animals: 37.1, Kidney of horse containing *K. equi* with young budding sporont (top), sporont with radiating sporoblasts (bottom left), and mature sporocysts (right) within tubular epithelium, X 250 (84-5266). 37.2, Epithelial cell of horse kidney tubule containing sporont of *K. equi*, with sporoblasts budding from central residual mass, X 630 (84-9461). 37.3, Kidney of horse with free sporoblasts of *K. equi* containing numerous nuclei, X 630 (84-5264). 37.4, Kidney of guinea pig infected with *K. cobayae*, X 250 (84-5257). 37.5, Epithelial cells of kidney tubule of guinea pig containing budding sporonts of *K. cobayae*, with sporoblasts budding from central residual mass, X 630 (84-5256). 37.6, Kidney of guinea pig with multinucleated sporocysts of *K. cobayae*, X 630 (84-5260).

Haemogregarina

Haemogregarina spp. are parasites of reptiles, amphibians, birds, and some mammals. They are transmitted to these hosts by invertebrates, such as leeches, ticks, mites, mosquitoes, and other hematophagous invertebrates. Invertebrates become infected by ingesting blood from an infected vertebrate host. When blood cells containing gamonts (CP38.3) are lysed in the gut of the invertebrate host, gametes fuse and an oocyst develops. This sporulates to form sporozoites, which are injected into the circulation of the vertebrate host during feeding or are ingested if the invertebrate host is eaten by the vertebrate.

Haemogregarine sporozoites infect erythrocytes of the vertebrate host, where they form trophozoites, and these grow into schizonts, which fill the cells. The enlarged erythrocytes containing the macroschizonts often appear to be extracellular in tissue sections (CP38.1, 38.2). Developing schizonts have nuclei at the periphery (CP38.1), and when mature the merozoites are crescent shaped (CP38.2). Merozoites released from the macroschizonts enter other erythrocytes and form a second generation, which, being smaller than the first generation, are termed microschizonts. Merozoites released from these enter erythrocytes and develop into either microgamonts or macrogametes. This ends development in the vertebrate host.

Hepatozoon

Hepatozoon spp. infect rodents, squirrels, canids, felids, raccoons, mink, and other carnivores, as well as birds and reptiles. Schizonts may be found in many visceral organs and the skeletal and heart muscles, but they are most common in the spleen and liver. *Hepatozoon* spp. are transmitted to vertebrate hosts by ticks, mites, lice, tsetse flies, mosquitoes, and other blood-sucking arthropods. The arthropods become infected by ingesting blood from an infected vertebrate host with gametocytes in leukocytes. Gametes released following digestion of leukocytes in the invertebrate gut undergo fertilization to form an ookinete, which undergoes sporogony to form sporozoites. When the invertebrate is ingested, sporozoites are released. They enter the bloodstream, are carried to the liver, and then leave the circulation and enter hepatic parenchymal cells, where they form schizonts. The schizonts, as in the *Haemogregarina* spp., at first have nuclei at the periphery (CP38.4). Later crescent-shaped merozoites bud from a residuum (CP38.5). Schizonts appear to be free in tissue sections but actually are intracellular in various visceral cells. Merozoites produced in schizonts reenter cells in the liver, producing at least three generations of schizonts. The final generation produces merozoites that enter mononuclear leukocytes and become microgamonts and macrogametes (CP38.6).

A wide spectrum of lesions has been reported, varying from very mild cellular infiltration to necrosis with accompanying cellular infiltration. Depending on the affected organ, extensive reticuloendothelial cell hyperplasia has also been reported.

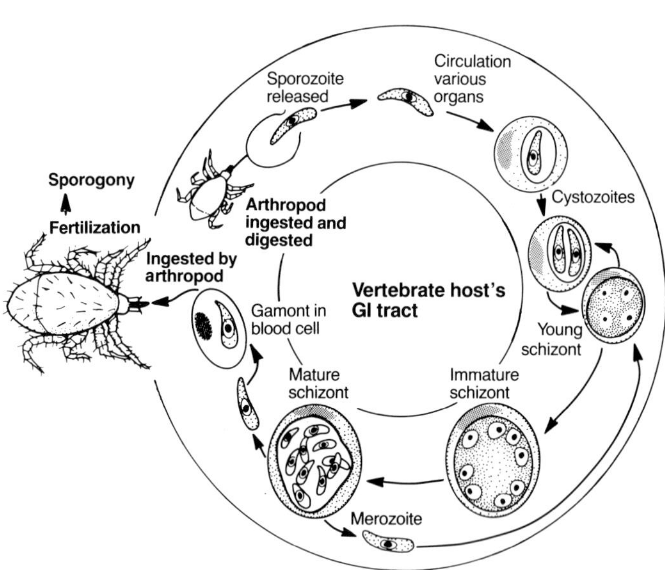

Hepatozoon

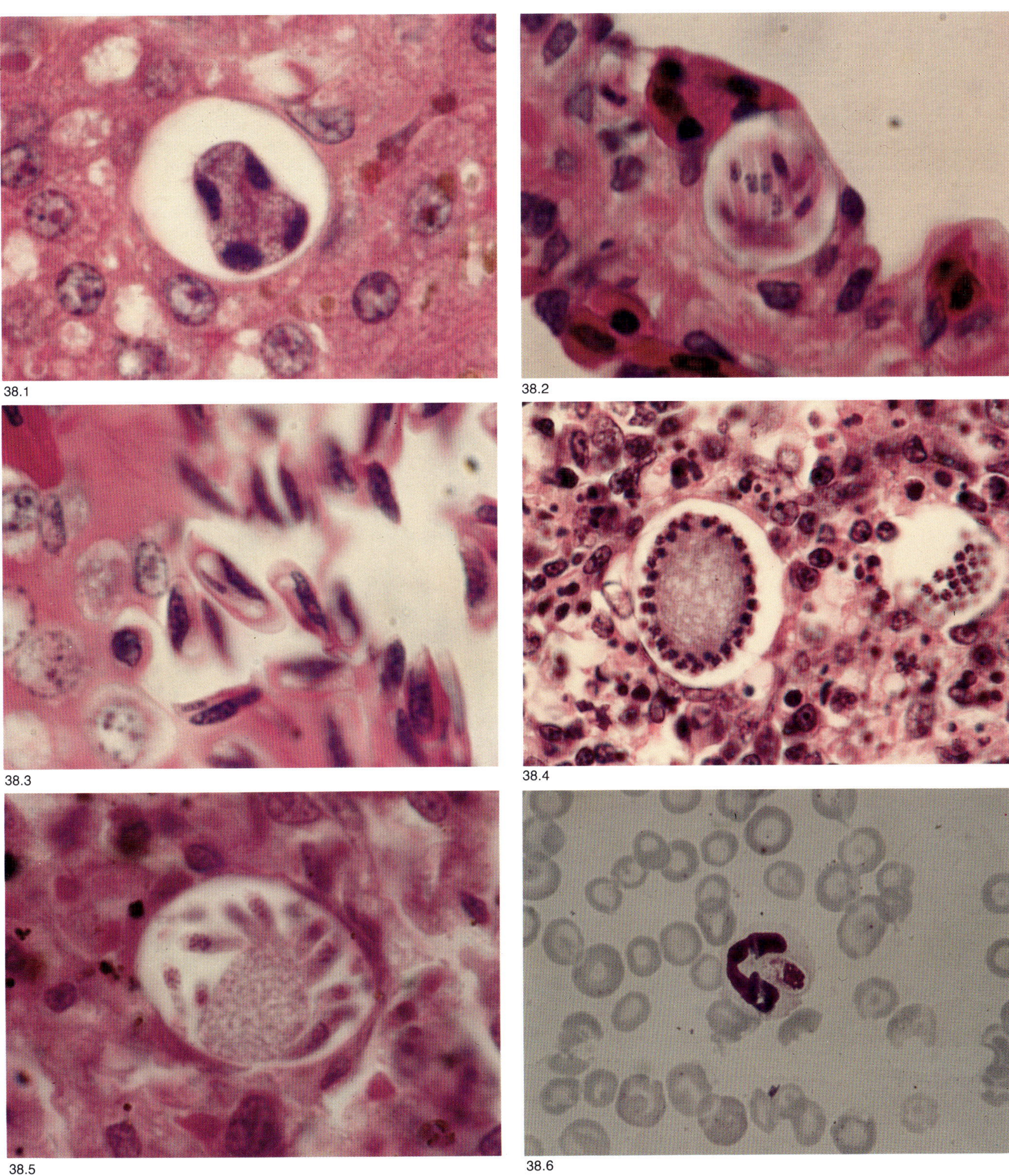

Color plate 38.—*Haemogregarina* sp. and *Hepatozoon canis* of animals: 38.1, Liver of boa constrictor containing developing schizont of *Haemogregarina* sp., X 1500 (84-9462). 38.2, Lung of boa constrictor containing schizont of *Haemogregarina* sp., X 1500 (84-9463). 38.3, Erythrocyte of boa constrictor containing macrogamete or microgamont of *Haemogregarina* sp., X 1500 (84-9464). 38.4, Spleen of dog containing developing schizont of *H. canis*, X 1000 (84-9465). 38.5, Spleen of dog containing schizont of *H. canis*; notice zoites budding from residual mass, X 1500 (84-9466). 38.6, Polymorphonuclear leucocyte of dog containing macrogamete or microgametocyte of *H. canis*, X 1500, Giemsa stain (84-5285).

Plasmodium

Plasmodium spp. infect most groups of higher vertebrates. Most are transmitted to vertebrate hosts by female mosquitoes. These and other arthropod hosts become infected by ingesting macrogametes and microgamonts in the blood of an infected vertebrate. In the invertebrate midgut, the latter form microgametes, which unite with the macrogametes to produce zygotes. The zygote transforms into a motile ookinete, which penetrates the gut wall and enters the coelom, where it develops into an oocyst. Oocysts undergo sporogony, producing thousands of sporozoites, which are injected into the vertebrate circulation when the invertebrate takes a blood meal. Sporozoites invade liver cells in most vertebrates, where they produce exoerythrocytic schizonts. This form multiplies asexually to produce tens of thousands of tissue-stage merozoites. Merozoites invade erythrocytes, where they transform into trophozoites (the feeding or ring stage) and multiply asexually to produce a schizont containing 8 to 32 erythrocytic merozoites. These merozoites invade other erythrocytes. The sexual phase begins when some merozoites in erythrocytes transform into macrogametes and microgamonts.

Gross lesions in severe malaria may include pallor caused by anemia, brown-tinged skin and mucous membranes due to malarial pigment, splenomegaly, and darkening of the viscera, especially liver, spleen, lungs, and brain, due to concentration of the pigment. Microscopic lesions are most obvious in the blood, where erythrocyte structure may be altered. During the blood phase of infection, there may be hypertrophy of Kupffer cells in the liver, with accumulation of malaria pigment, interlobular inflammation, and glycogen depletion followed by fatty infiltration. In the kidneys, there may be pigment accumulation in macrophages and parasites in erythrocytes in veins, fatty degeneration of the parenchyma, and possibly immune complex glomerulonephritis. In the lungs, there may be accumulation of pigment in macrophages in the capillaries, obstruction of the vasculature and lymphatics, and pulmonary edema. In the spleen, there may be hyperplasia of red and white pulp (primarily lymphocytes and macrophages), congestion, and erythrophagocytosis.

Diagnosis is primarily by thick or thin blood smears. Intraerythrocytic organisms stained with Giemsa are red (chromatin), blue (cytoplasm), and yellow to black (pigment) (CP 39.1-39.3, 40.1).

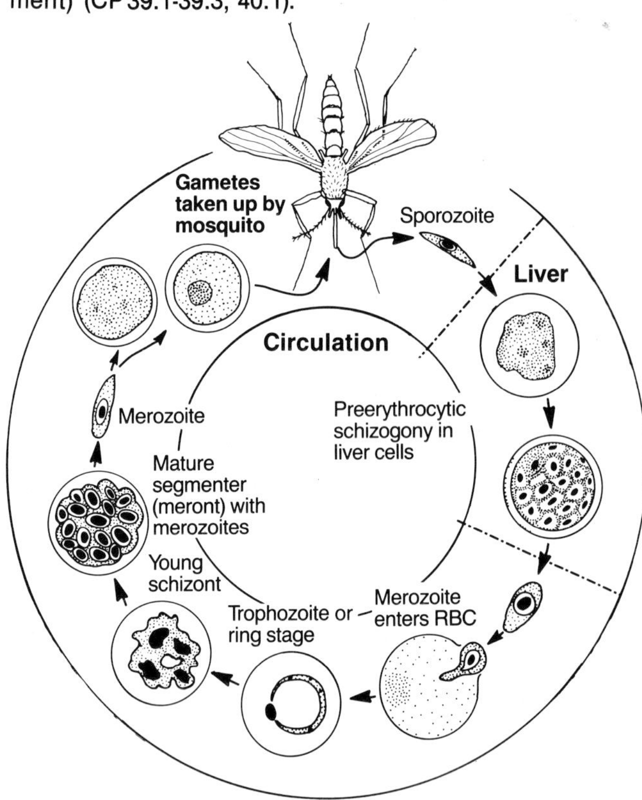

Plasmodium

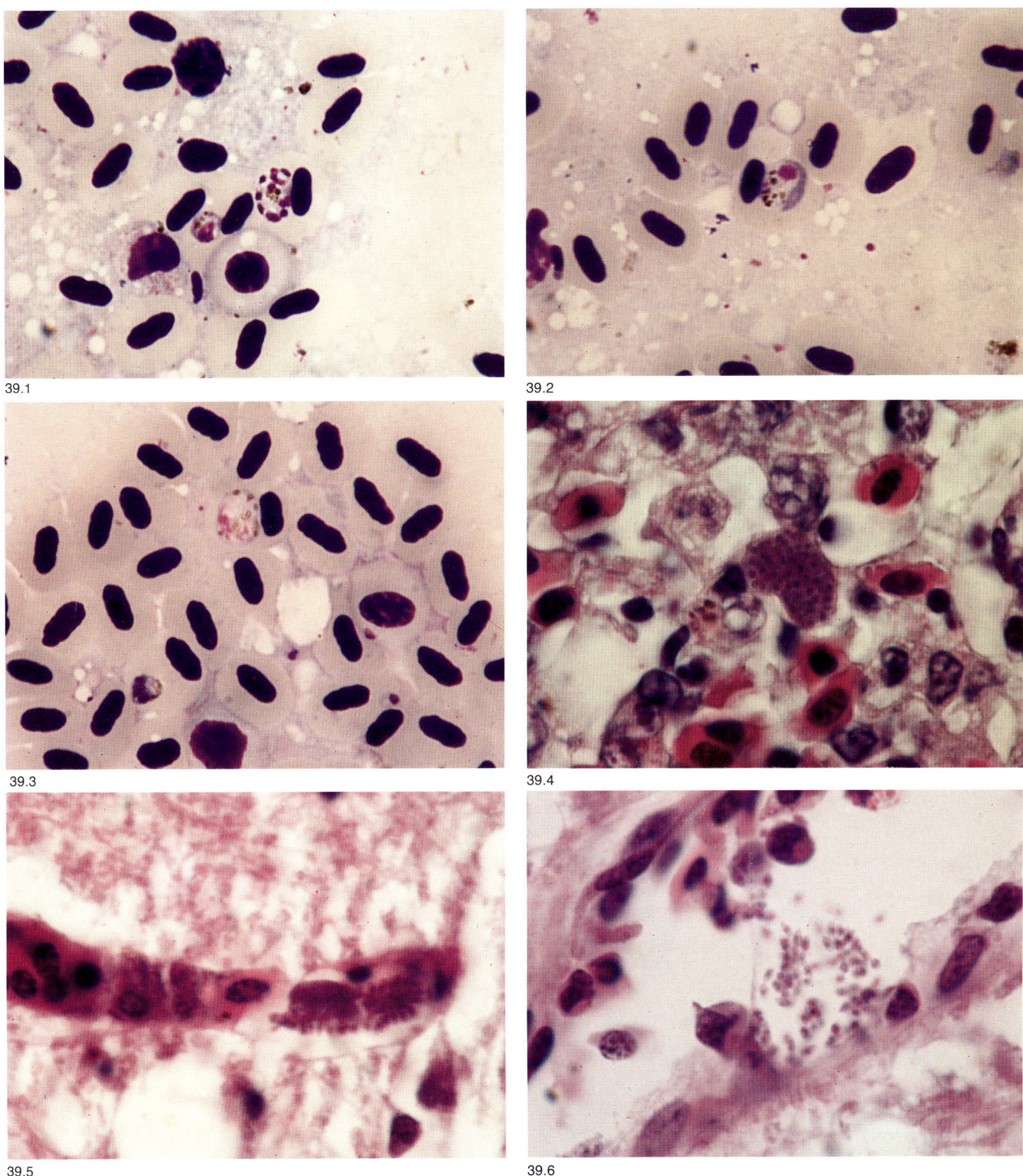

Color plate 39.—*Plasmodium* spp. of birds: 39.1, Blood smear from starling; note schizont (right, center) of *P. relictum* with numerous nuclei, X 1500, Giemsa stain (84-9467). 39.2, Blood smear from starling with macrogamete of *P. relictum*, X 1500, Giemsa stain (84-9468). 39.3, Blood smear from starling with gamont of *P. relictum*, X 1500, Giemsa stain (84-9472). 39.4, Lung of penguin with exoerythrocytic schizont of *Plasmodium* sp., X 1500 (84-9469). 39.5, Endothelial cell of turkey brain with exoerythrocytic schizont of *P. durae*, X 1500 (84-9470). 39.6, Endothelium of turkey brain with merozoites being released from schizont of *P. durae*, X 1500 (84-9471).

Hepatocystis

Hepatocystis spp. parasitize arboreal tropical mammals of the Old World, especially squirrels, fruit bats, and lower monkeys, as well as deer mice and the hippopotamus. Sporozoites, inoculated into the circulation during feeding by the vector (*Culicoides* spp.), enter the hepatic parenchymal cells of the mammals and develop into meronts. These meronts, termed merocysts, may reach 4-6 mm in diameter (CP40.4-40.6). As the merocysts enlarge, a big vacuole forms in the center and fills with colloid (CP40.4). Merozoites develop at the periphery of the merocyst. When merocysts mature in 1 or 2 months, they rupture and release merozoites, which invade erythrocytes and resemble the ring stage of *Plasmodium* spp. (CP40.2). Multinucleate bodies are also released from the merocysts occasionally. They enter the circulation and are called "corps plasmatiques." Their function is not known. Microgamonts and macrogametes develop in erythrocytes. After ingestion of blood containing gametocytes by the invertebrate host, microgametes are formed, and fertilization and sporogony take place.

Lesions observed microscopically are usually limited to inflammatory cells around merocysts.

Differentiation of *Hepatocystis* spp. from other hemoproteid parasites is based on structure and staining characteristics. For example, when stained with Giemsa, microgamonts of *Hepatocystis* have an unusual nucleus, with a large, oval, pink nucleoplasm that occupies one-third or more of the parasite. Within the nucleus are numerous red chromatin granules or threads.

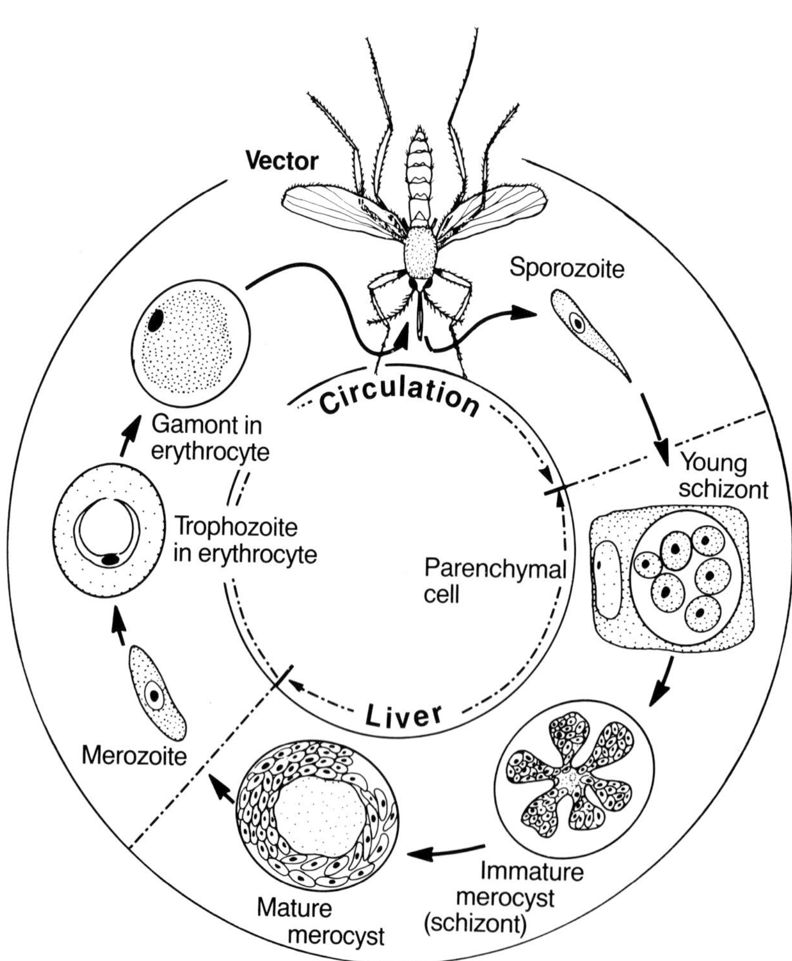

Hepatocystis

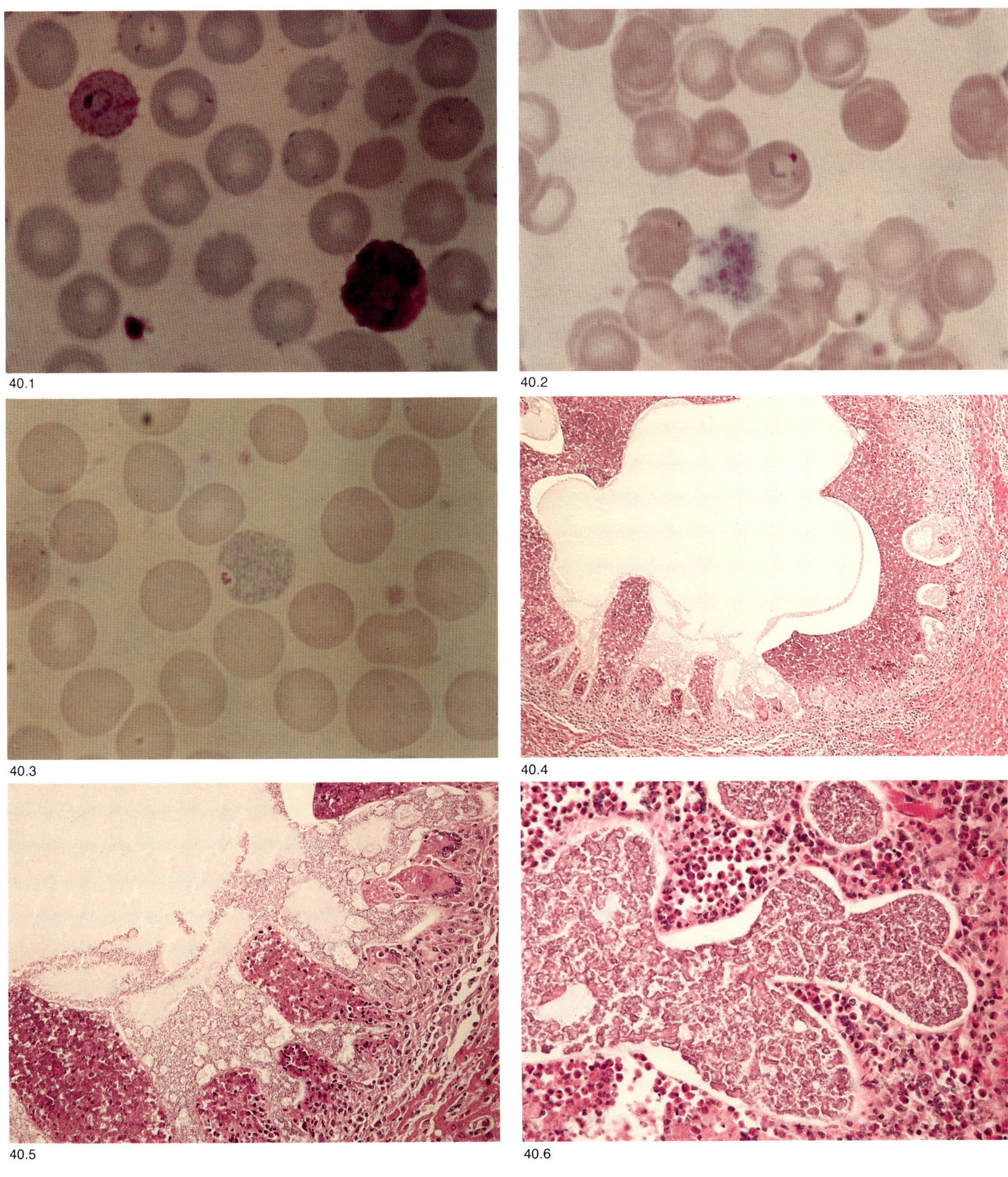

40.1

40.2

40.3

40.4

40.5

40.6

Color plate 40.—*Plasmodium* sp. and *Hepatocystis* sp. of nonhuman primates: 40.1, Blood smear from monkey showing trophozoite (left) and schizont (right) of *P. cynomolgi,* X 1500, Giemsa stain (84-9473). 40.2, Blood smear from monkey with trophozoite of *Hepatocystis* sp., X 1500, Giemsa stain (84-9474). 40.3, Blood smear from monkey with macrogamete of *Hepatocystis* sp., X 1500, Giemsa stain (84-9475). 40.4, Liver of monkey with merocyst of *Hepatocystis* sp., X 60 (84-9476). 40.5, Higher magnification of merocyst showing formation of merozoites, X 160 (84-9477). 40.6, Still higher magnification of merozoite formation in wall of merocyst, X 250 (84-9478).

Theileria (Syn., Cytauxzoon)

Theileria has been reported among domestic and wild
ungulates in southern Africa and in wild and domestic
felids in several States in the United States. Domestic
cats are thought to be accidental hosts. Ticks are the
vectors. Intraerythrocytic stages (trophozoites) may be
absent or present in the circulating blood. They vary in
structure from round to oval with an eccentric nucleus,
or they may be elongate with bipolar chromatin bodies.
Schizonts (meronts) are found in leukocytes,
erythroblasts, histiocytic macrophages, and other host
cells. Developing schizonts have numerous large
vesicular nuclei (CP 41.2-41.4), whereas mature
schizonts contain myriads of uninucleate merozoites
with small nuclei (CP41.4, 41.5). Merozoites released
from schizonts invade erythrocytes (CP41.6).

The most characteristic lesion is the occlusion of the
lumen of medium and small blood vessels and
sinusoids in organs, including the heart, liver, lung,
lymph nodes, kidney, and spleen, with large schizont-
containing macrophages (CP41.1).

Theileria spp. are diagnosed in mammalian tissues as
schizonts in leukocytes, macrophages, and other cells
and as trophozoites in erythrocytes (CP41.6).

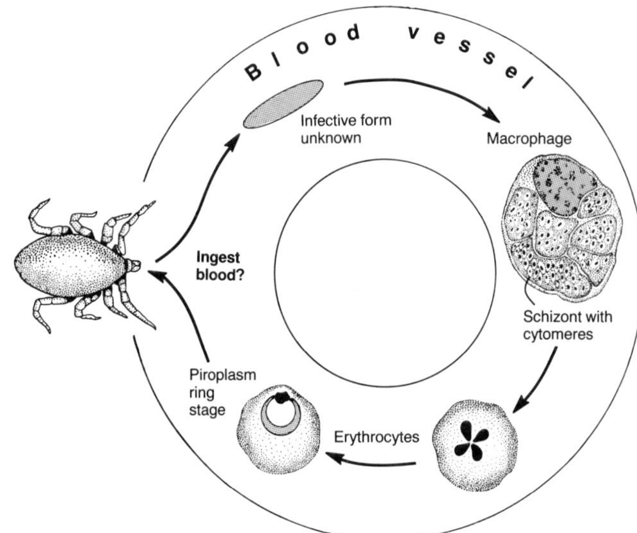

Theileria

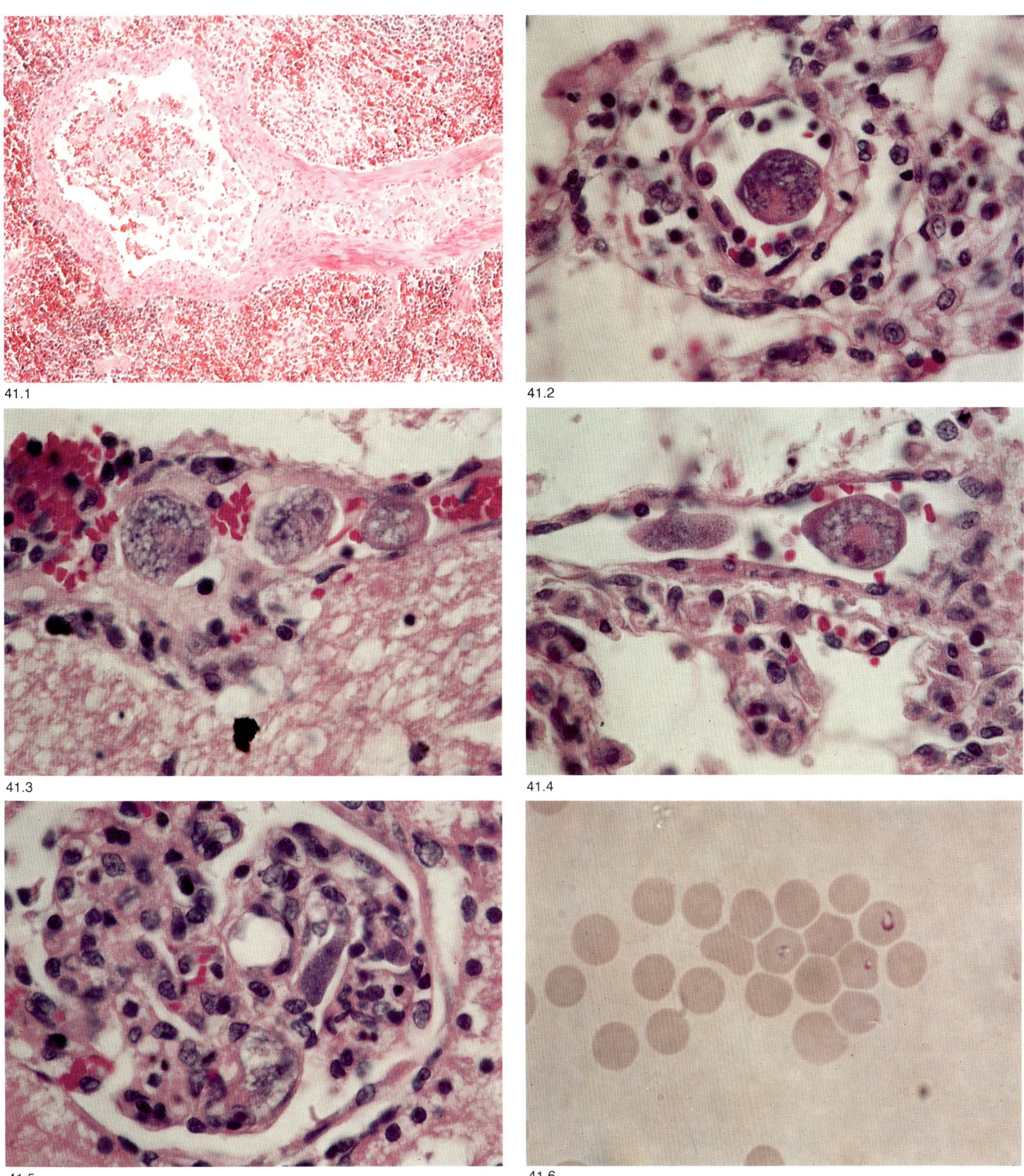

41.1

41.2

41.3

41.4

41.5

41.6

Color plate 41.—*Theileria felis* (syn., *Cytaux-zoon felis*) of cats: 41.1, Splenic artery with schizonts of *T. felis* occluding lumen, X 100 (84-9485).   41.2, Macrophage containing schizont of *T. felis* that seems to bud from endothelium of pulmonary vein, X 630 (84-5278). 41.3, Pulmonary vessel with three developing schizonts of *T. felis,* X 630 (84-5284).   41.4, Pulmonary vessel with developing and mature (left) schizonts of *T. felis,* X 630 (84-5283).   41.5, Capillary of glomerulus with schizont of *T. felis,* X 630 (84-5282). 41.6, Blood smear with trophozoites of *T. felis* in erythrocytes, X 1500 (84-9486).

Babesia

Babesia spp. infect domestic animals, including cattle, sheep, goats, horses, swine, dogs, and cats, as well as numerous wild animals (nearly 70 species) and man. Some *Babesia* spp. are not host specific and can be transmitted among mammalian hosts. After inoculation by a tick vector, *Babesia* spp. enter the bloodstream and multiply asexually by schizogony in erythrocytes. Stages of development elsewhere in the body have not been identified. Intraerythrocytic *Babesia* spp. are seen singly as round, ovoid, elongate, or amoeboid trophozoites, in pairs as pyriform merozoites, or in tetrads as cruciform merozoites. Ticks become infected by ingesting infected blood. Sexual stages of *Babesia* have not been identified, but large motile vermicules develop in the tick and migrate throughout the body undergoing an unknown number of generations of schizogony. Vermicules produced by schizogony eventually infect tick eggs, multiply in the yolk, and continue to multiply in tissues of the larva, eventually causing small pyriform bodies in the salivary cells. These infect the mammalian host.

Although there are widespread differences in pathogenicity among members of this genus and numerous clinical signs, the primary lesion based on studies in cattle is erythrocyte destruction. Microscopically during the acute hemolytic phase of anemia, erythrocytes are normocytic. They later become macrocytic and reticulocytes appear. The liver may undergo centrilobular and midzonal necrosis, with hemosiderin deposits in Kupffer cells and phagocytosis of erythrocytes. The kidneys may be congested in the interlobular capillaries with many infected erythrocytes; tubular epithelium may have large deposits of hemosiderin and may degenerate; and casts may form. Lungs, heart, spleen, lymph nodes, and brain may be congested and capillaries distended with infected erythrocytes.

Microscopic examination of peripheral blood smears is the basic diagnostic procedure for the acute disease (CP42.1-42.3). *Babesia* spp. are best diagnosed in thick and thin smears stained with Giemsa. Differentiation from *Anaplasma* (CP42.4), *Ehrlichia* (CP42.5), and *Theileria* (CP41.6) is based on the structure of the blood stages. *Anaplasma* spp. are tiny (1 μm) intraerythrocytic spheres. *Ehrlichia* spp. are found singly and in clumps within circulating monocytes or granulocytes. *Theileria* spp. are found as multinucleate Koch's blue bodies (macroschizonts) in lymphocytes and as micro-merozoites, gamonts, and gametes in erythrocytes. Forms in erythrocytes are often called small piroplasms (1.2-2.5 μm) to differentiate them from the larger piroplasms of *Babesia*. Diverse shapes (elongate, bacillary-like, or bayonet-like) are further characteristics of *Theileria*.

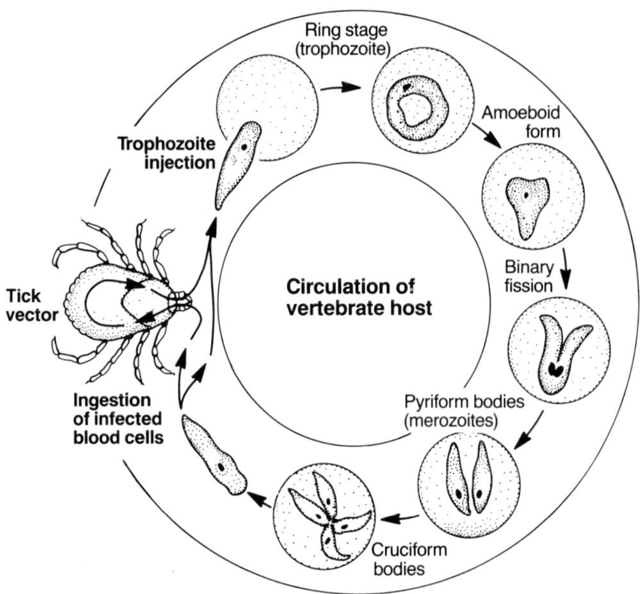

Babesia

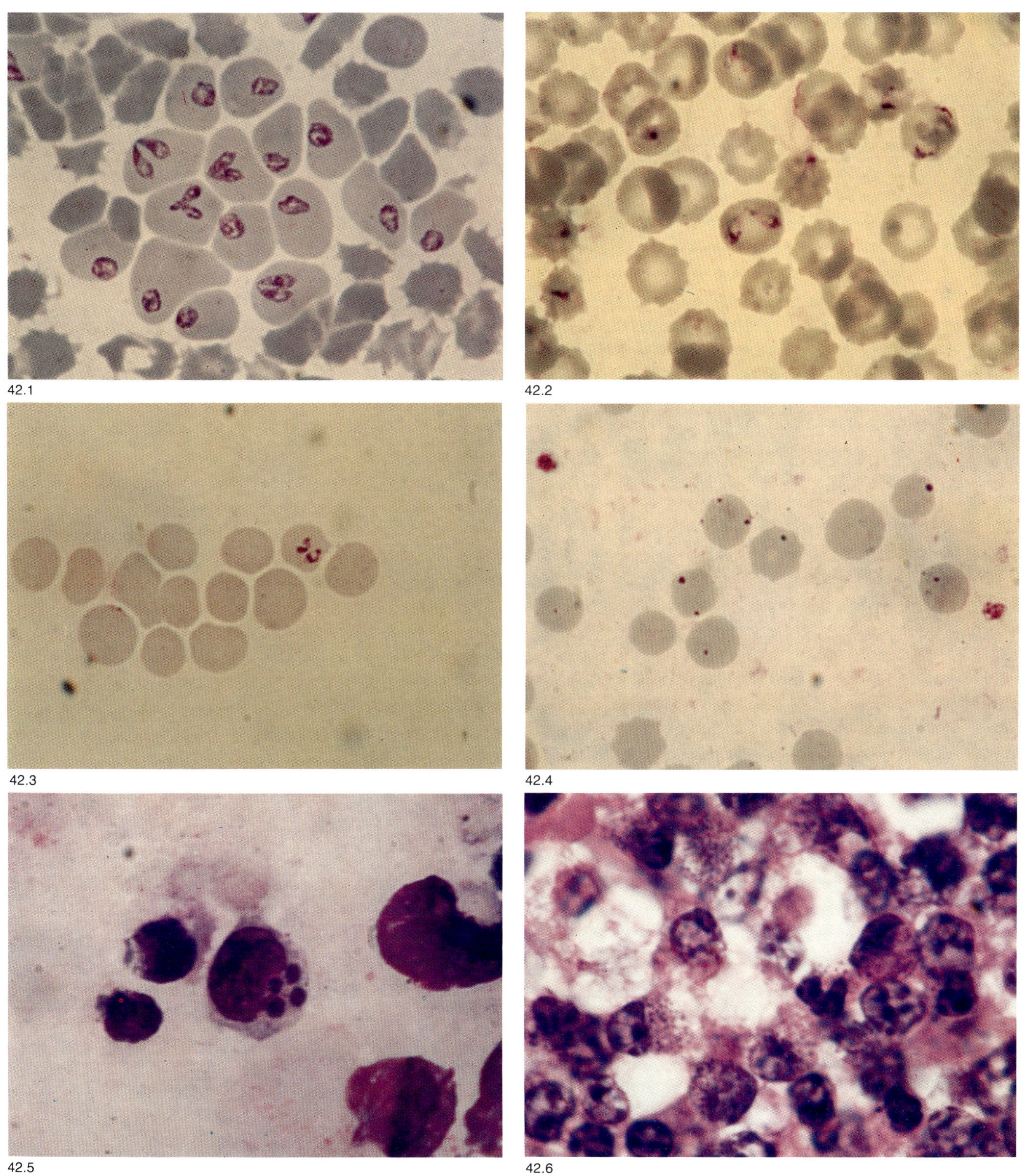

Color plate 42.—Piroplasms and rickettsiae of animals: 42.1, Peripheral blood smear of pig with intraerythrocytic *Babesia trautmanni*, X 1500, Neitz stain (84-9479). 42.2, Peripheral blood smear of dog with intraerythrocytic *B. canis*, X 1500, Giemsa stain (84-9480). 42.3, Peripheral blood smear of horse with intraerythrocytic *B. caballi*, X 1500, Giemsa stain (84-9481). 42.4, Peripheral blood smear of horse with intraerythrocytic *Anaplasma marginale*, X 1500, Giemsa stain (84-9482). 42.5, Peripheral blood smear of dog with intraleucocytic *Ehrlichia canis*, X 1500, Neitz stain (84-9483). 42.6, Lymphocytes within lymph node of cow containing intracellular *Theileria parva*, X 1500 (84-9484).

Haemoproteus

Haemoproteus spp. are found primarily in birds; some parasitize turtles and lizards. Of over 80 named species, many are indistinguishable from one another, are named on the basis of the host in which they are found, and have incompletely known life histories. All species have insect vectors, such as midges, hipposcids, or tabanids. Sporozoites in the salivary glands of the insect vector are thought to enter the circulation of the vertebrate host when the insect bites. The first stage seen in vertebrates is the elongate, twisted schizont in the vascular endothelium of the lung (CP43.1, 43.2), liver, kidney, and spleen. Merozoites develop within the schizont in clusters. When mature, they are released into the circulation as tiny (1-2 μm) round bodies. They enter erythrocytes (CP43.3), where they transform into macrogametes or microgamonts, the only stages seen in the insect after ingestion of infected blood.

Parasitemia exceeding 50 percent of erythrocytes has been observed without signs of disease.

Diagnosis is primarily based on identification of microgamonts or macrogametes in blood smears or of schizonts in smears or sections of organs.

Leucocytozoon

Leucocytozoon spp. are found in birds. Of over 70 named species, many are indistinguishable from one another; they are named because of being found in different host species. Their life histories are incompletely known. All species have insect vectors, such as midges and simuliid flies. Sporozoites in the salivary gland of the insect enter the circulation of the bird when the insect bites. First generation schizonts of most species then develop in hepatic parenchymal cells and when mature release thousands of tiny (1 μm) round merozoites that are thought to initiate a second generation in hepatic parenchymal and phagocytic cells throughout the body. Those in phagocytic cells usually become very large (100-200 μm) megaloschizonts (CP43.4). When mature, they release millions of tiny (1 μm) round merozoites that either initiate schizogony in hepatic parenchymal cells or enter circulating erythrocytes or leukocytes, where they develop into microgamonts or macrogametes. Those of some species are exclusively round (CP43.5), and those of other species are thought to be round at one time and elongate (CP43.6) at another. Sexual maturation, fertilization, and sporogony take place in the insect after ingestion of infected blood.

For those species of *Leucocytozoon* that are pathogenic, the basic lesion is destruction of erythrocytes resulting in anemia. Inflammatory and necrotic foci may be found in the liver.

Diagnosis is primarily based on identification of gamonts or gametes in blood smears or of megaloschizonts in smears or sections of organs.

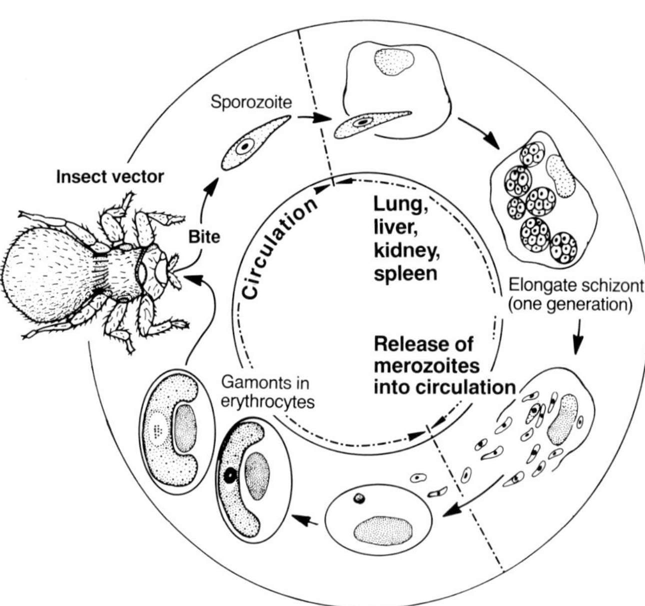

Haemoproteus

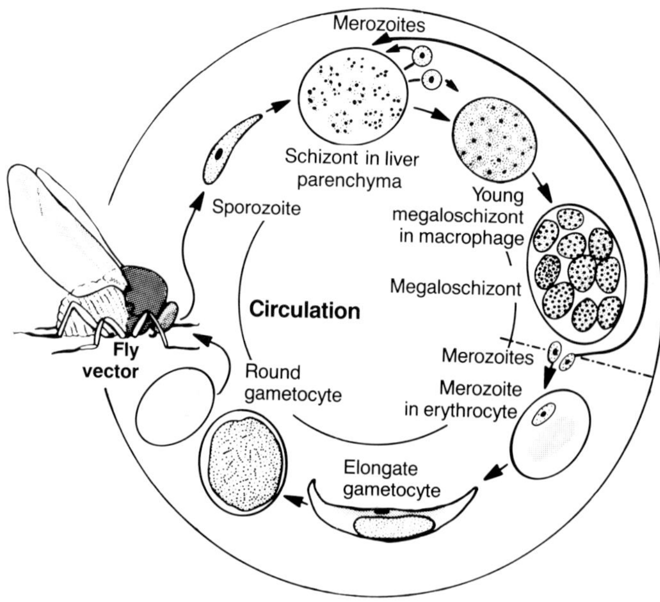

Leucocytozoon

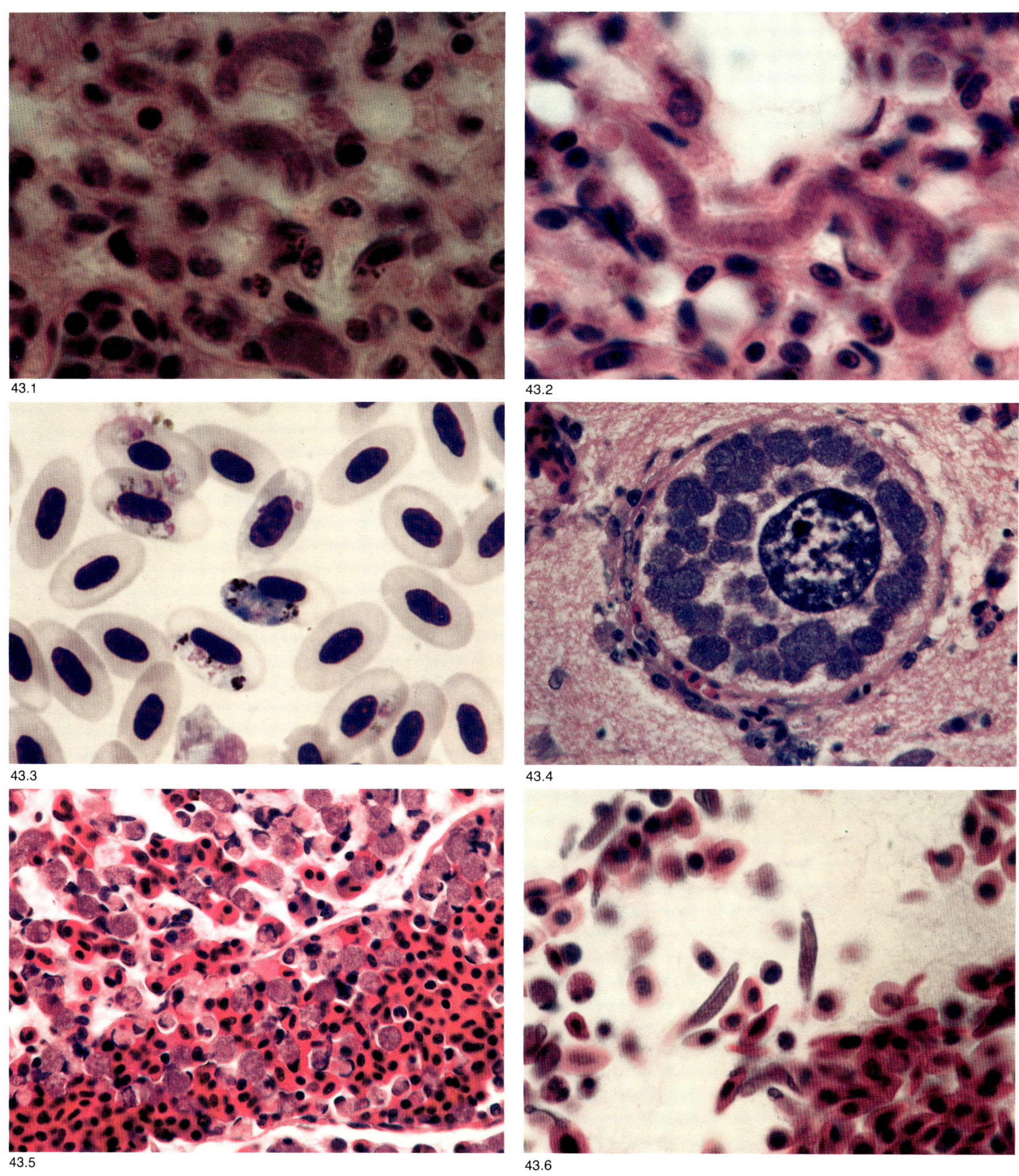

Color plate 43.—Haemosporozoa of birds: 43.1, Lung of pigeon with numerous schizonts of *Haemoproteus* sp., X 1500 (84-5291).   43.2, Lung of pigeon with sinuous schizont of *Haemoproteus* sp., X 1500 (84-9487).   43.3, Blood smear from pigeon with merozoites (small organisms) and larger microgamonts or macrogametes of *Haemoproteus* sp. within erythrocytes, X 1500, Giemsa stain (84-9488).   43.4, Brain of duck with megaloschizont of *Leucocytozoon simondi* in cell with distinct hypertrophied nucleus, X 630 (84-5300).   43.5, Lung of robin with round microgamonts or macrogametes of *Leucocytozoon* sp. in erythrocytes, X 630 (84-9489).   43.6, Liver of duck with elongate microgamonts or macrogametes of *Leucocytozoon* sp. in erythrocytes, X 1000 (84-9490).

Large "cysts" of haemosporozoa have been reported from the gizzard, skeletal and cardiac muscles, and visceral organs of a variety of birds (CP44.1, 44.2). In these reports, gamonts and gametes have not been found in peripheral blood smears. In some cysts the contents are compartmentalized by internal septa (CP44.3-44.5). Hemorrhage is sometimes associated with cysts, and blood cells appear within or among groups of organisms (CP44.5, 44.6).

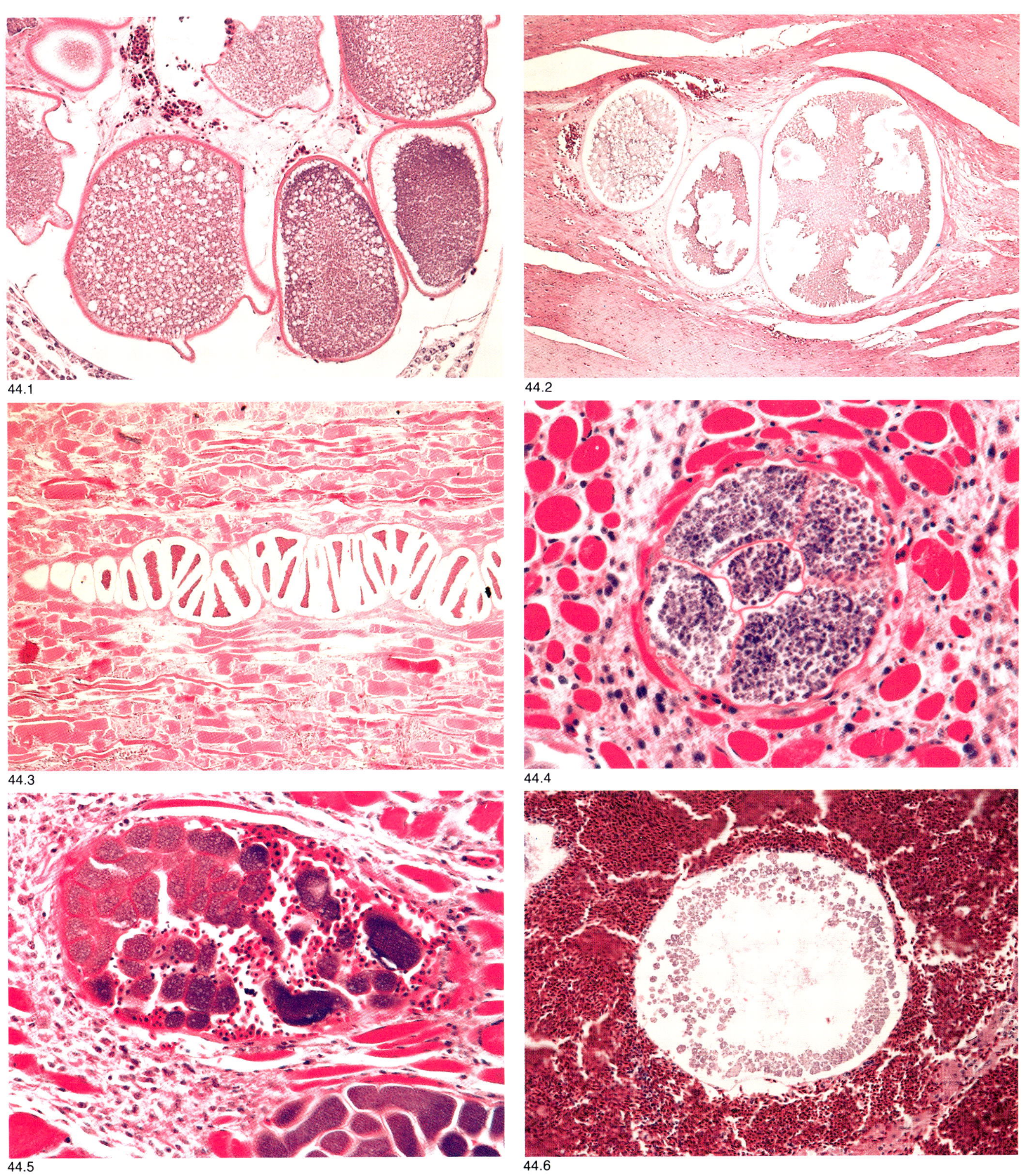

Color plate 44.—Haemosporozoa of birds: 44.1, Pancreas of chicken with schizonts of *Leucocytozoon caulleryi* (syn., *Akiba caulleryi*), X 160 (84-9491). 44.2, Gizzard of parakeet with schizonts of *Leucocytozoon*-like organism, X 60 (84-9492). 44.3, Skeletal muscle of curawong with schizont of *Leucocytozoon*-like organism, X 60 (84-9493). 44.4, Muscle of quail with compartmentalized cyst of haemosporozoan, X 400 (84-9494). 44.5, Muscle of quail showing compartmentalized cyst of haemosporozoan with erythrocytes scattered among compartments, X 250 (84-9495). 44.6, Liver of pigeon containing cyst of haemosporozoan with organisms at periphery and large empty central area, X 160 (84-9496).

Fungi

Some genera of fungi are often mistaken for protozoans.
Diphasic fungi develop as yeasts in animal tissues and
are often difficult to identify. Yeast forms of
Histoplasma capsulatum and *Candida albicans* (CP45)
are similar to amastigotes of *Leishmania* spp. (CP1.2)
and *Trypanosoma cruzi* (CP1.5, 1.6). Some fungi form
spores or sporangia that resemble protozoan cysts. For
example, spores of *Emmonsia* spp. (CP47) resemble
thick-walled cysts of some haemosporozoans (CP44),
sporangia of *Coccidioides* and *Prototheca* (CP48) are
similar to sarcocysts of *Sarcocystis* (CP24), yeasts of
Blastomyces and *Loboa* (CP50) resemble various stages
of coccidia (CP31, 36), and sporangia of *Rhinosporidium* spp. (CP46) are like megaloschizonts of
Leucocytozoon spp. (CP43.4).

Special stains, such as Gomori methanamine silver,
periodic acid-Schiff reaction, Gridley fungus, and
mucicarmine, are necessary to differentiate fungi from
protozoans. Fungi commonly found in animal tissues
are illustrated in color plates 45-50.

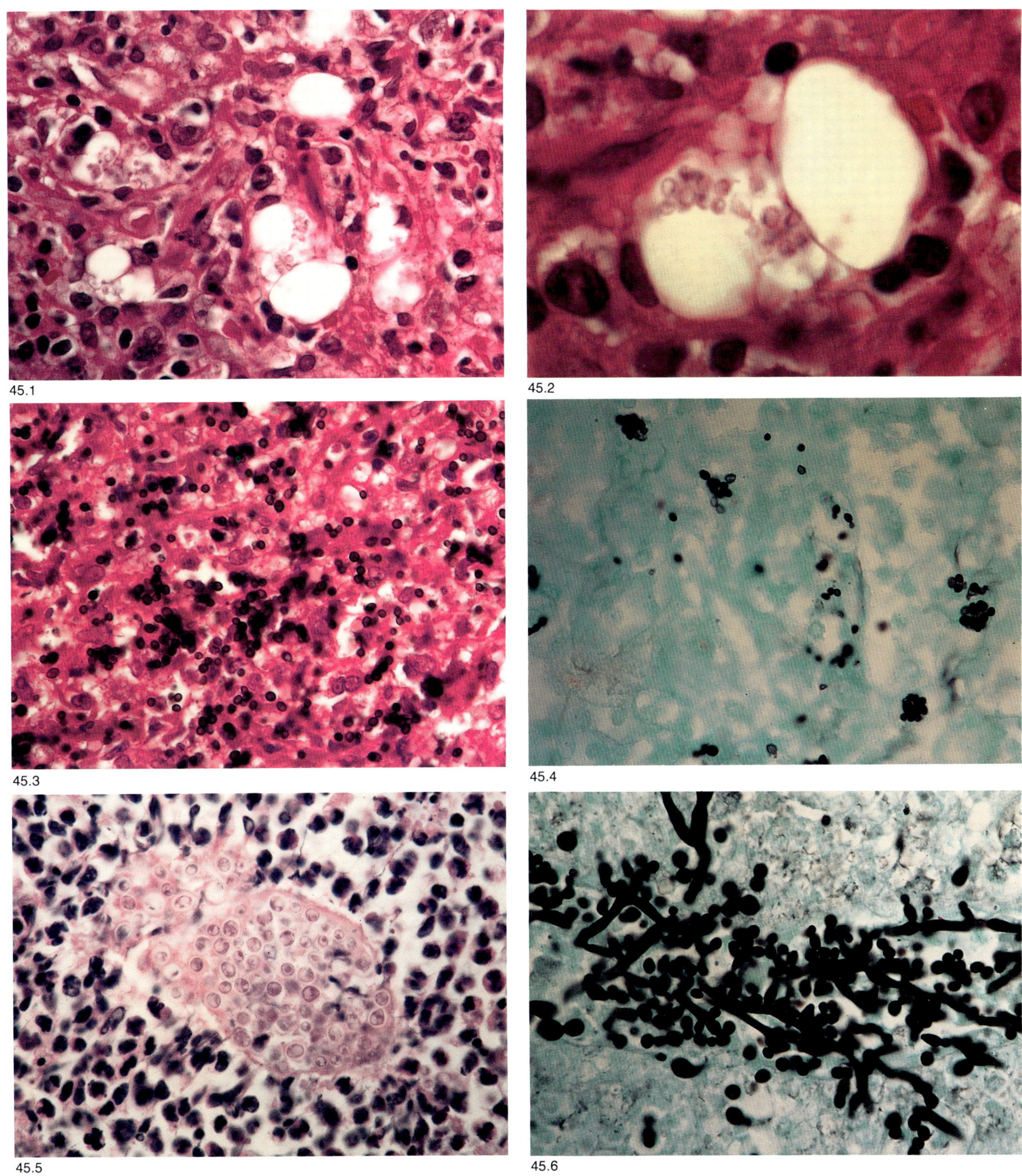

45.1

45.2

45.3

45.4

45.5

45.6

Color plate 45.—*Histoplasma capsulatum* and *Candida albicans* of animals: 45.1, Skin of dog with vacuoles within macrophages containing small (2-4 μm) yeast forms of *H. capsulatum*, X 630 (84-9583). 45.2, Skin of dog at higher magnification with organisms resembling amastigotes of *Leishmania* spp. (CP1.2), X 1500 (84-9584). 45.3, Skin of dog with *Histoplasma* stained with silver and easily identified in this photomicrograph, X 630, Gomori methanamine silver (GMS) with H&E counterstain (84-9585). 45.4, Lung of dog with *Histoplasma* stained with silver, X 630, GMS stain (84-9586). 45.5, Kidney of killer whale with numerous small (3-7 μm) yeasts of *C. albicans* faintly stained and resembling amastigotes of *Leishmania* spp., X 630 (84-9587). 45.6, Kidney of killer whale with yeasts and pseudohyphae of *Candida* readily seen, X 630, GMS stain (84-9588).

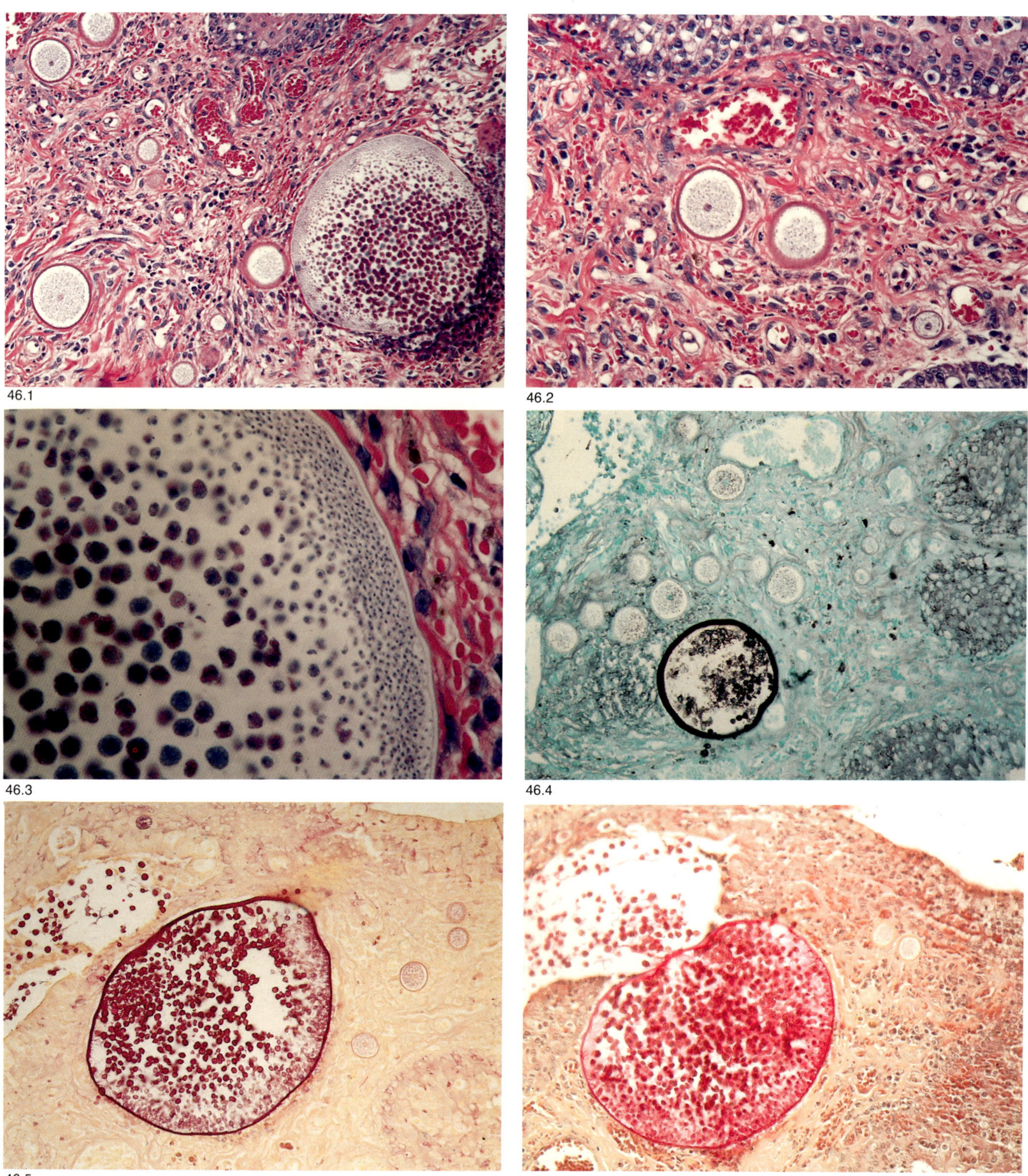

Color plate 46.—*Rhinosporidium seeberi* of dogs: 46.1, Nasal polyp; note larger mature sporangium (right) and smaller trophic stages throughout stroma, X 160 (84-9589). 46.2, Nasal polyp containing trophic stage with thick wall and some with one large nucleus, X 250 (84-9590). 46.3, Nasal polyp with thick, somewhat hyaline wall of mature sporangium containing young (periphery of cyst) and mature spores (center of cyst) with eosinophilic globules; sporangium resembles megaloschizont of *Leucocytozoon* spp. (CP43.4), X 630 (84-9591). 46.4, Nasal polyp with Gomori methanamine silver stained wall of mature sporangium and spores within, but trophic stages not stained, X 160, GMS stain (84-9592). 46.5, Nasal polyp containing mature sporangium and spores within are stained bright pink, X 160, Gridley fungus stain (84-9593). 46.6, Nasal polyp with mature ruptured sporangium releasing spores into lumen of nasal cavity, X 160, mucicarmine stain (84-9594).

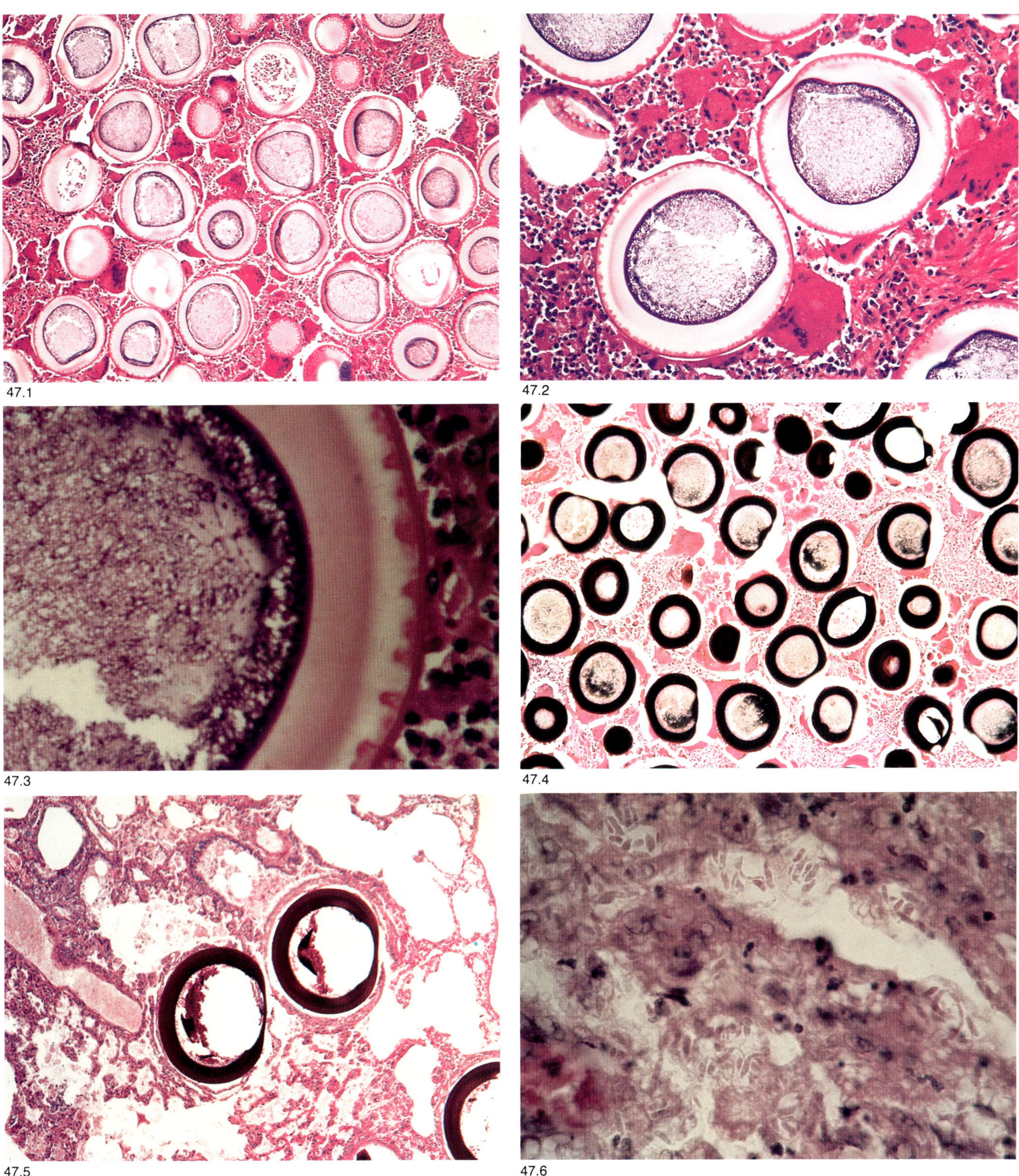

Color plate 47.—*Emmonsia crescens* and *Sporothrix schenckii* of animals: 47.1, Peritoneum of monkey with numerous thick-walled adiaspores of *E. crescens* resembling cysts of *Besnoitia* (CP29.1-29.3), X 60 (84-9595). 47.2, Peritoneum of monkey at higher magnification of adiaspores of *E. crescens,* X 160 (84-9596). 47.3, Peritoneum of monkey at still higher magnification of adiaspore wall of *E. crescens*, X 630 (84-9597). 47.4, Peritoneum of monkey with walls of adiaspores of *E. crescens* stained black, X 60, GMS stain (84-9598). 47.5, Lung of water rat (*Arvicola* sp.) with black walls of *E. crescens*, X 60, GMS stain (84-9599). 47.6, Leg of cat with subcutaneous mass containing numerous elongate yeasts of *S. schenckii*, X 640 (84-9600).

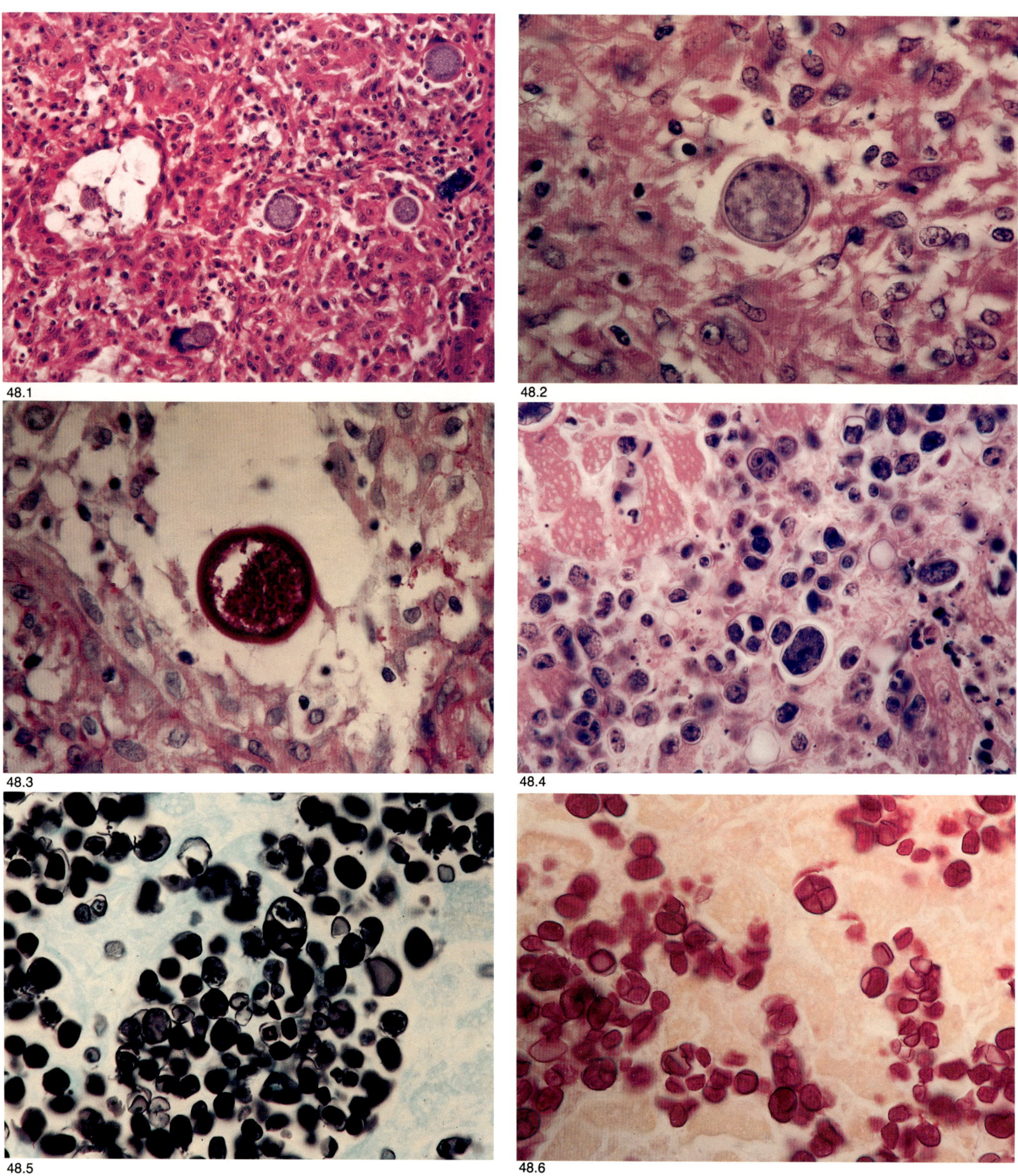

Color plate 48.—*Coccidioides immitis* and *Prototheca* sp. of animals: 48.1, Liver of sea lion with oval, basophilic sporangia of *C. immitis* resembling sarcocysts of *Sarcocystis*, X 250 (84-9601).   48.2, Pericardium of dog containing developing sporangium of *C. immitis* with thick, hyaline wall and multiple nuclei surrounding basophilic cytoplasm, X 630 (84-9602).   48.3, Pericardium of dog with mature sporangia containing endospores stained bright red, X 630, PAS stain (84-9603).   48.4, Heart of dog containing stages of *Prototheca* sp. with achlorophyllous mutant of green algae, with large parent cells (sporangia) containing numerous smaller progeny cells, each with its own thick cell wall, X 630 (84-9604). 48.5, Heart of dog with several parent cells (sporangia) of *Prototheca* sp. containing up to four progeny cells, X 630, GMS stain (84-9605).   48.6, Heart of dog with several sporangia of *Prototheca* sp., X 630, Gridley fungus stain (84-9606).

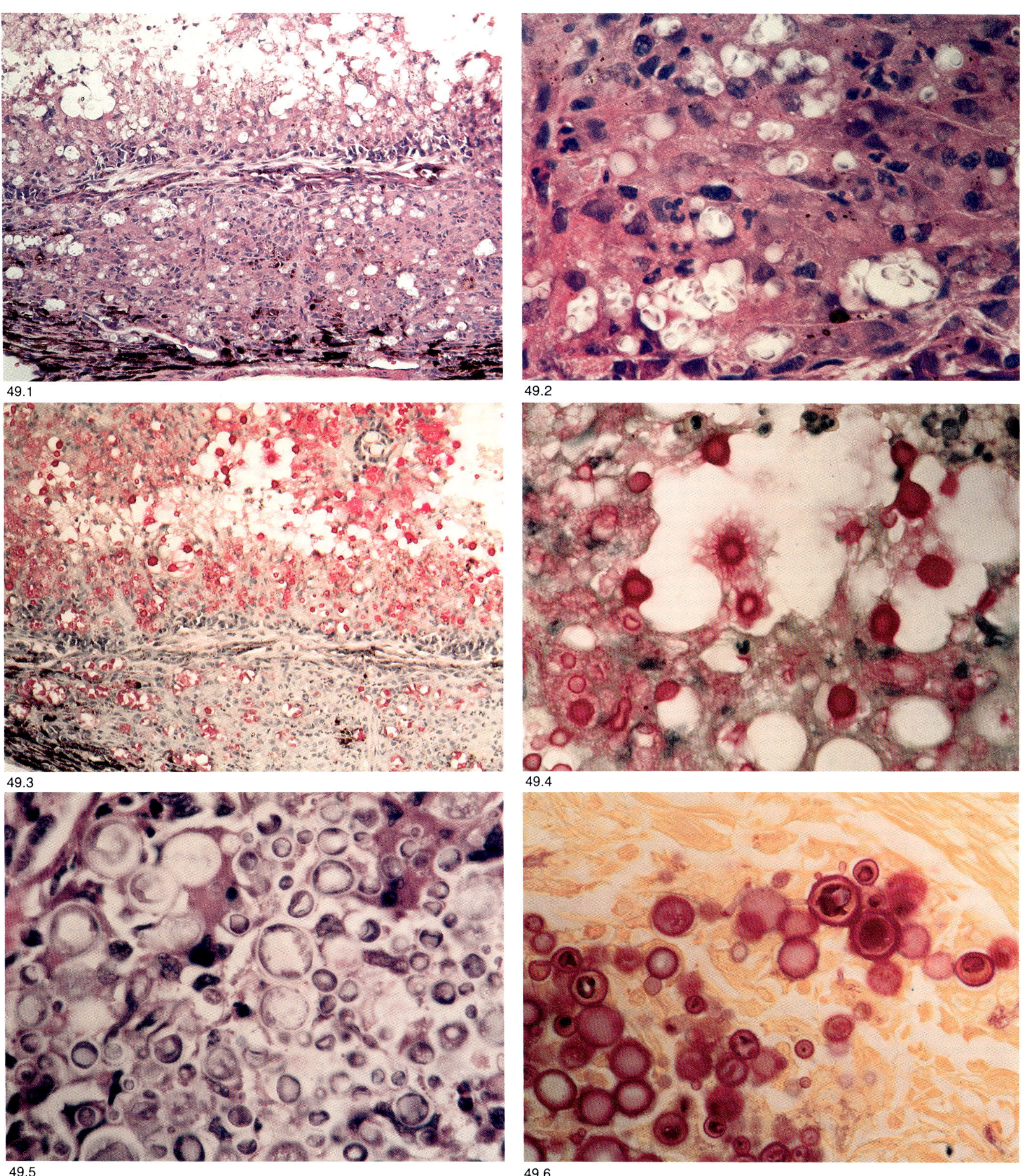

Color plate 49.—*Cryptococcus neoformans* and *Paracoccidioides brasiliensis* of animals: 49.1, Eye of dog with numerous faintly stained yeasts of *C. neoformans* within inflammatory mass, X 160 (84-9607).   49.2, Eye of dog at higher magnification, X 630 (84-9608).   49.3, Eye of dog with mucinous capsules of yeasts of *C. neoformans* stained brilliant pink, X 160, mucicarmine stain (84-9609).   49.4, Eye of dog at higher magnification, X 630, mucicarmine stain (84-9610).   49.5, Liver of monkey with numerous various sized yeasts (5-15 μm) of *P. brasiliensis*, X 630 (84-9611).   49.6, Liver of monkey containing large yeast of *P. brasiliensis* (top right) with characteristic multiple budding, X 630, Gridley fungus stain (84-9612).

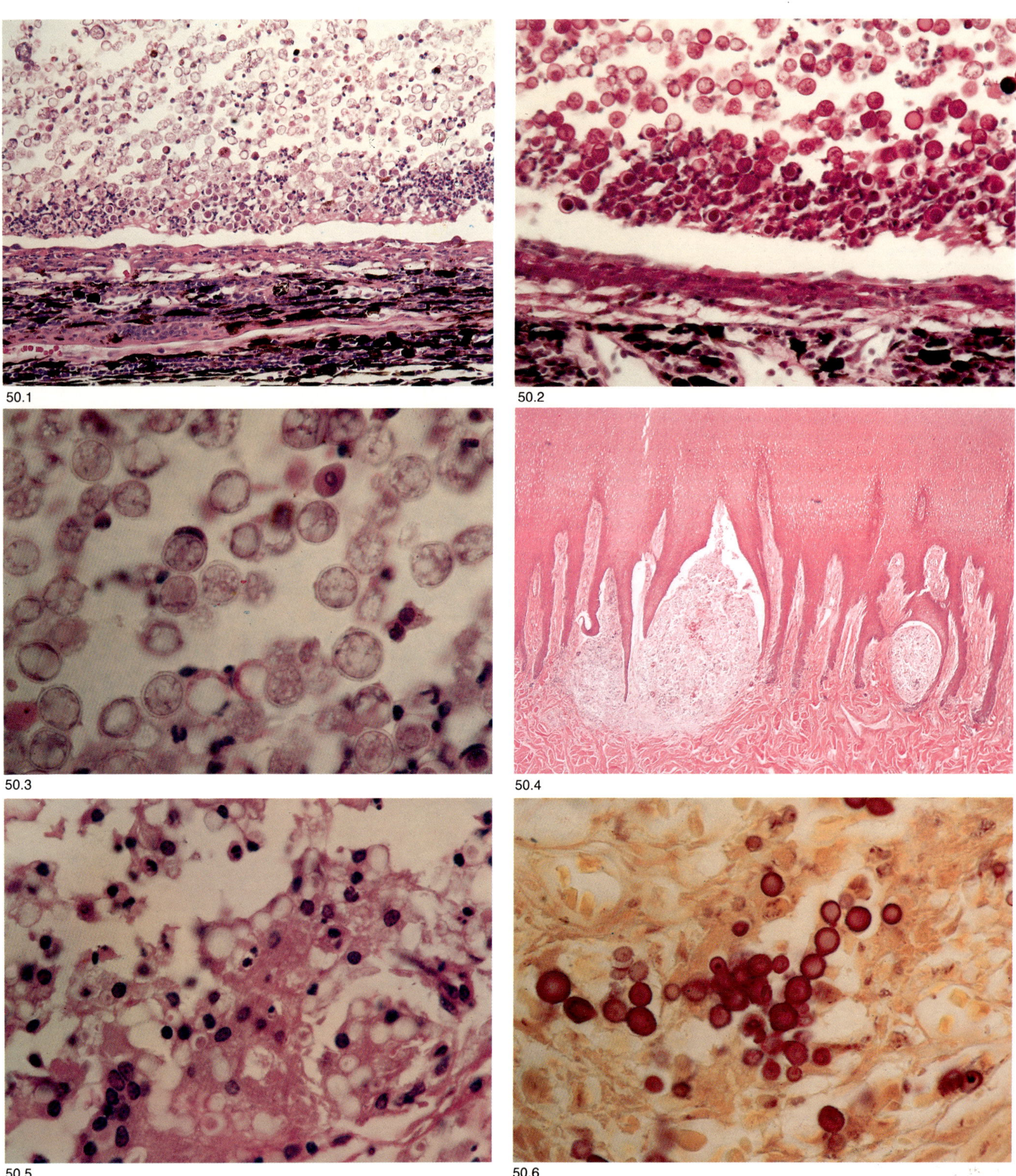

Color plate 50.—*Blastomyces dermatitidis* and *Loboa loboi* of animals: 50.1, Eye of dog with numerous yeasts of *B. dermatitidis* within inflammatory mass, X 160 (84-9613). 50.2, Eye of dog with yeasts of *B. dermatitidis* stained red, X 250, PAS stain (84-9614). 50.3, Eye of dog containing yeasts of *B. dermatitidis* with thick walls and multiple nuclei within foamy cytoplasm, X 630 (84-9615). 50.4, Skin of dolphin with inflammatory masses in dermis due to yeasts of *L. loboi*, X 25 (84-9616). 50.5, Skin of dolphin with yeasts of *L. loboi* faintly stained and appearing to form chains, X 630 (84-9617). 50.6, Skin of dolphin with characteristic chain of *L. loboi*, X 630, Gridley fungus stain (84-9618).

DATE DUE